FREE Study Skills DVD Offer

Dear Customer,

Thank you for your purchase from Mometrix! We consider it an honor and a privilege that you have purchased our product and we want to ensure your satisfaction.

As a way of showing our appreciation and to help us better serve you, we have developed a Study Skills DVD that we would like to give you for FREE. This DVD covers our *best practices* for getting ready for your exam, from how to use our study materials to how to best prepare for the day of the test.

All that we ask is that you email us with feedback that would describe your experience so far with our product. Good, bad, or indifferent, we want to know what you think!

To get your FREE Study Skills DVD, email freedvd@mometrix.com with *FREE STUDY SKILLS DVD* in the subject line and the following information in the body of the email:

- The name of the product you purchased.
- Your product rating on a scale of 1-5, with 5 being the highest rating.
- Your feedback. It can be long, short, or anything in between. We just want to know your impressions and experience so far with our product. (Good feedback might include how our study material met your needs and ways we might be able to make it even better. You could highlight features that you found helpful or features that you think we should add.)
- Your full name and shipping address where you would like us to send your free DVD.

If you have any questions or concerns, please don't hesitate to contact me directly.

Thanks again!

Sincerely,

Jay Willis
Vice President
jay.willis@mometrix.com
1-800-673-8175

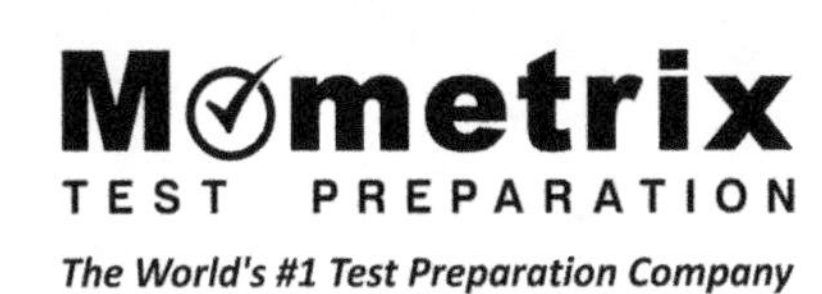

Registered Dietitian Exam SECRETS

Study Guide

Your Key to Exam Success

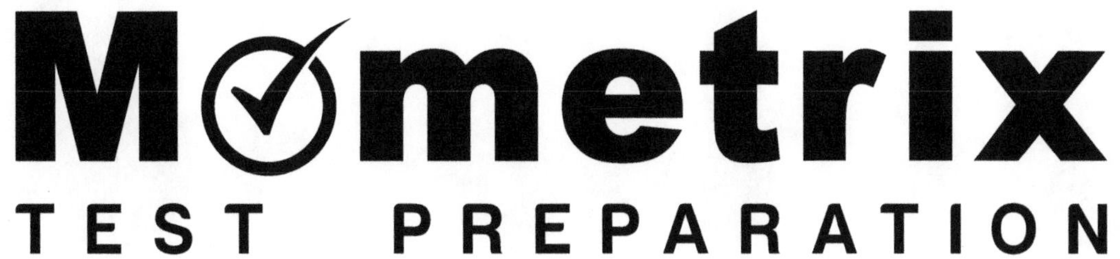

Written and edited by the Mometrix Dietitian Certification Test Team

Mometrix offers volume discount pricing to institutions. For more information or a price quote, please contact our sales department at sales@mometrix.com or 888-248-1219.

Paperback
ISBN 13: 978-1-61072-803-4
ISBN 10: 1-61072-803-3

Ebook
ISBN 13: 978-1-62120-455-8
ISBN 10: 1-62120-455-3

Hardback
ISBN 13: 978-1-5167-0555-9
ISBN 10: 1-5167-0555-6

Dear Future Exam Success Story

First of all, **THANK YOU** for purchasing Mometrix study materials!

Second, congratulations! You are one of the few determined test-takers who are committed to doing whatever it takes to excel on your exam. **You have come to the right place.** We developed these study materials with one goal in mind: to deliver you the information you need in a format that's concise and easy to use.

In addition to optimizing your guide for the content of the test, we've outlined our recommended steps for breaking down the preparation process into small, attainable goals so you can make sure you stay on track.

We've also analyzed the entire test-taking process, identifying the most common pitfalls and showing how you can overcome them and be ready for any curveball the test throws you.

Standardized testing is one of the biggest obstacles on your road to success, which only increases the importance of doing well in the high-pressure, high-stakes environment of test day. Your results on this test could have a significant impact on your future, and this guide provides the information and practical advice to help you achieve your full potential on test day.

Your success is our success

We would love to hear from you! If you would like to share the story of your exam success or if you have any questions or comments in regard to our products, please contact us at **800-673-8175** or **support@mometrix.com**.

Thanks again for your business and we wish you continued success!

Sincerely,
The Mometrix Test Preparation Team

TABLE OF CONTENTS

Introduction

Thank you for purchasing this resource! You have made the choice to prepare yourself for a test that could have a huge impact on your future, and this guide is designed to help you be fully ready for test day. Obviously, it's important to have a solid understanding of the test material, but you also need to be prepared for the unique environment and stressors of the test, so that you can perform to the best of your abilities.

For this purpose, the first section that appears in this guide is the **Secret Keys**. We've devoted countless hours to meticulously researching what works and what doesn't, and we've boiled down our findings to the five most impactful steps you can take to improve your performance on the test. We start at the beginning with study planning and move through the preparation process, all the way to the testing strategies that will help you get the most out of what you know when you're finally sitting in front of the test.

We recommend that you start preparing for your test as far in advance as possible. However, if you've bought this guide as a last-minute study resource and only have a few days before your test, we recommend that you skip over the first two Secret Keys since they address a long-term study plan.

If you struggle with **test anxiety**, we strongly encourage you to check out our recommendations for how you can overcome it. Test anxiety is a formidable foe, but it can be beaten, and we want to make sure you have the tools you need to defeat it.

Secret Key #1 – Plan Big, Study Small

There's a lot riding on your performance. If you want to ace this test, you're going to need to keep your skills sharp and the material fresh in your mind. You need a plan that lets you review everything you need to know while still fitting in your schedule. We'll break this strategy down into three categories.

Information Organization

Start with the information you already have: the official test outline. From this, you can make a complete list of all the concepts you need to cover before the test. Organize these concepts into groups that can be studied together, and create a list of any related vocabulary you need to learn so you can brush up on any difficult terms. You'll want to keep this vocabulary list handy once you actually start studying since you may need to add to it along the way.

Time Management

Once you have your set of study concepts, decide how to spread them out over the time you have left before the test. Break your study plan into small, clear goals so you have a manageable task for each day and know exactly what you're doing. Then just focus on one small step at a time. When you manage your time this way, you don't need to spend hours at a time studying. Studying a small block of content for a short period each day helps you retain information better and avoid stressing over how much you have left to do. You can relax knowing that you have a plan to cover everything in time. In order for this strategy to be effective though, you have to start studying early and stick to your schedule. Avoid the exhaustion and futility that comes from last-minute cramming!

Study Environment

The environment you study in has a big impact on your learning. Studying in a coffee shop, while probably more enjoyable, is not likely to be as fruitful as studying in a quiet room. It's important to keep distractions to a minimum. You're only planning to study for a short block of time, so make the most of it. Don't pause to check your phone or get up to find a snack. It's also important to **avoid multitasking**. Research has consistently shown that multitasking will make your studying dramatically less effective. Your study area should also be comfortable and well-lit so you don't have the distraction of straining your eyes or sitting on an uncomfortable chair.

The time of day you study is also important. You want to be rested and alert. Don't wait until just before bedtime. Study when you'll be most likely to comprehend and remember. Even better, if you know what time of day your test will be, set that time aside for study. That way your brain will be used to working on that subject at that specific time and you'll have a better chance of recalling information.

Finally, it can be helpful to team up with others who are studying for the same test. Your actual studying should be done in as isolated an environment as possible, but the work of organizing the information and setting up the study plan can be divided up. In between study sessions, you can discuss with your teammates the concepts that you're all studying and quiz each other on the details. Just be sure that your teammates are as serious about the test as you are. If you find that your study time is being replaced with social time, you might need to find a new team.

Secret Key #2 – Make Your Studying Count

You're devoting a lot of time and effort to preparing for this test, so you want to be absolutely certain it will pay off. This means doing more than just reading the content and hoping you can remember it on test day. It's important to make every minute of study count. There are two main areas you can focus on to make your studying count:

Retention

It doesn't matter how much time you study if you can't remember the material. You need to make sure you are retaining the concepts. To check your retention of the information you're learning, try recalling it at later times with minimal prompting. Try carrying around flashcards and glance at one or two from time to time or ask a friend who's also studying for the test to quiz you.

To enhance your retention, look for ways to put the information into practice so that you can apply it rather than simply recalling it. If you're using the information in practical ways, it will be much easier to remember. Similarly, it helps to solidify a concept in your mind if you're not only reading it to yourself but also explaining it to someone else. Ask a friend to let you teach them about a concept you're a little shaky on (or speak aloud to an imaginary audience if necessary). As you try to summarize, define, give examples, and answer your friend's questions, you'll understand the concepts better and they will stay with you longer. Finally, step back for a big picture view and ask yourself how each piece of information fits with the whole subject. When you link the different concepts together and see them working together as a whole, it's easier to remember the individual components.

Finally, practice showing your work on any multi-step problems, even if you're just studying. Writing out each step you take to solve a problem will help solidify the process in your mind, and you'll be more likely to remember it during the test.

Modality

Modality simply refers to the means or method by which you study. Choosing a study modality that fits your own individual learning style is crucial. No two people learn best in exactly the same way, so it's important to know your strengths and use them to your advantage.

For example, if you learn best by visualization, focus on visualizing a concept in your mind and draw an image or a diagram. Try color-coding your notes, illustrating them, or creating symbols that will trigger your mind to recall a learned concept. If you learn best by hearing or discussing information, find a study partner who learns the same way or read aloud to yourself. Think about how to put the information in your own words. Imagine that you are giving a lecture on the topic and record yourself so you can listen to it later.

For any learning style, flashcards can be helpful. Organize the information so you can take advantage of spare moments to review. Underline key words or phrases. Use different colors for different categories. Mnemonic devices (such as creating a short list in which every item starts with the same letter) can also help with retention. Find what works best for you and use it to store the information in your mind most effectively and easily.

Secret Key #3 – Practice the Right Way

Your success on test day depends not only on how many hours you put into preparing, but also on whether you prepared the right way. It's good to check along the way to see if your studying is paying off. One of the most effective ways to do this is by taking practice tests to evaluate your progress. Practice tests are useful because they show exactly where you need to improve. Every time you take a practice test, pay special attention to these three groups of questions:

- The questions you got wrong
- The questions you had to guess on, even if you guessed right
- The questions you found difficult or slow to work through

This will show you exactly what your weak areas are, and where you need to devote more study time. Ask yourself why each of these questions gave you trouble. Was it because you didn't understand the material? Was it because you didn't remember the vocabulary? Do you need more repetitions on this type of question to build speed and confidence? Dig into those questions and figure out how you can strengthen your weak areas as you go back to review the material.

Additionally, many practice tests have a section explaining the answer choices. It can be tempting to read the explanation and think that you now have a good understanding of the concept. However, an explanation likely only covers part of the question's broader context. Even if the explanation makes sense, **go back and investigate** every concept related to the question until you're positive you have a thorough understanding.

As you go along, keep in mind that the practice test is just that: practice. Memorizing these questions and answers will not be very helpful on the actual test because it is unlikely to have any of the same exact questions. If you only know the right answers to the sample questions, you won't be prepared for the real thing. **Study the concepts** until you understand them fully, and then you'll be able to answer any question that shows up on the test.

It's important to wait on the practice tests until you're ready. If you take a test on your first day of study, you may be overwhelmed by the amount of material covered and how much you need to learn. Work up to it gradually.

On test day, you'll need to be prepared for answering questions, managing your time, and using the test-taking strategies you've learned. It's a lot to balance, like a mental marathon that will have a big impact on your future. Like training for a marathon, you'll need to start slowly and work your way up. When test day arrives, you'll be ready.

Start with the strategies you've read in the first two Secret Keys—plan your course and study in the way that works best for you. If you have time, consider using multiple study resources to get different approaches to the same concepts. It can be helpful to see difficult concepts from more than one angle. Then find a good source for practice tests. Many times, the test website will suggest potential study resources or provide sample tests.

Practice Test Strategy

If you're able to find at least three practice tests, we recommend this strategy:

Untimed and Open-Book Practice

Take the first test with no time constraints and with your notes and study guide handy. Take your time and focus on applying the strategies you've learned.

Timed and Open-Book Practice

Take the second practice test open-book as well, but set a timer and practice pacing yourself to finish in time.

Timed and Closed-Book Practice

Take any other practice tests as if it were test day. Set a timer and put away your study materials. Sit at a table or desk in a quiet room, imagine yourself at the testing center, and answer questions as quickly and accurately as possible.

Keep repeating timed and closed-book tests on a regular basis until you run out of practice tests or it's time for the actual test. Your mind will be ready for the schedule and stress of test day, and you'll be able to focus on recalling the material you've learned.

Secret Key #4 – Pace Yourself

Once you're fully prepared for the material on the test, your biggest challenge on test day will be managing your time. Just knowing that the clock is ticking can make you panic even if you have plenty of time left. Work on pacing yourself so you can build confidence against the time constraints of the exam. Pacing is a difficult skill to master, especially in a high-pressure environment, so **practice is vital**.

Set time expectations for your pace based on how much time is available. For example, if a section has 60 questions and the time limit is 30 minutes, you know you have to average 30 seconds or less per question in order to answer them all. Although 30 seconds is the hard limit, set 25 seconds per question as your goal, so you reserve extra time to spend on harder questions. When you budget extra time for the harder questions, you no longer have any reason to stress when those questions take longer to answer.

Don't let this time expectation distract you from working through the test at a calm, steady pace, but keep it in mind so you don't spend too much time on any one question. Recognize that taking extra time on one question you don't understand may keep you from answering two that you do understand later in the test. If your time limit for a question is up and you're still not sure of the answer, mark it and move on, and come back to it later if the time and the test format allow. If the testing format doesn't allow you to return to earlier questions, just make an educated guess; then put it out of your mind and move on.

On the easier questions, be careful not to rush. It may seem wise to hurry through them so you have more time for the challenging ones, but it's not worth missing one if you know the concept and just didn't take the time to read the question fully. Work efficiently but make sure you understand the question and have looked at all of the answer choices, since more than one may seem right at first.

Even if you're paying attention to the time, you may find yourself a little behind at some point. You should speed up to get back on track, but do so wisely. Don't panic; just take a few seconds less on each question until you're caught up. Don't guess without thinking, but do look through the answer choices and eliminate any you know are wrong. If you can get down to two choices, it is often worthwhile to guess from those. Once you've chosen an answer, move on and don't dwell on any that you skipped or had to hurry through. If a question was taking too long, chances are it was one of the harder ones, so you weren't as likely to get it right anyway.

On the other hand, if you find yourself getting ahead of schedule, it may be beneficial to slow down a little. The more quickly you work, the more likely you are to make a careless mistake that will affect your score. You've budgeted time for each question, so don't be afraid to spend that time. Practice an efficient but careful pace to get the most out of the time you have.

Secret Key #5 – Have a Plan for Guessing

When you're taking the test, you may find yourself stuck on a question. Some of the answer choices seem better than others, but you don't see the one answer choice that is obviously correct. What do you do?

The scenario described above is very common, yet most test takers have not effectively prepared for it. Developing and practicing a plan for guessing may be one of the single most effective uses of your time as you get ready for the exam.

In developing your plan for guessing, there are three questions to address:

- When should you start the guessing process?
- How should you narrow down the choices?
- Which answer should you choose?

When to Start the Guessing Process

Unless your plan for guessing is to select C every time (which, despite its merits, is not what we recommend), you need to leave yourself enough time to apply your answer elimination strategies. Since you have a limited amount of time for each question, that means that if you're going to give yourself the best shot at guessing correctly, you have to decide quickly whether or not you will guess.

Of course, the best-case scenario is that you don't have to guess at all, so first, see if you can answer the question based on your knowledge of the subject and basic reasoning skills. Focus on the key words in the question and try to jog your memory of related topics. Give yourself a chance to bring the knowledge to mind, but once you realize that you don't have (or you can't access) the knowledge you need to answer the question, it's time to start the guessing process.

It's almost always better to start the guessing process too early than too late. It only takes a few seconds to remember something and answer the question from knowledge. Carefully eliminating wrong answer choices takes longer. Plus, going through the process of eliminating answer choices can actually help jog your memory.

Summary: Start the guessing process as soon as you decide that you can't answer the question based on your knowledge.

How to Narrow Down the Choices

The next chapter in this book (**Test-Taking Strategies**) includes a wide range of strategies for how to approach questions and how to look for answer choices to eliminate. You will definitely want to read those carefully, practice them, and figure out which ones work best for you. Here though, we're going to address a mindset rather than a particular strategy.

Your chances of guessing an answer correctly depend on how many options you are choosing from.

How many choices you have	How likely you are to guess correctly
5	20%
4	25%
3	33%
2	50%
1	100%

You can see from this chart just how valuable it is to be able to eliminate incorrect answers and make an educated guess, but there are two things that many test takers do that cause them to miss out on the benefits of guessing:

- Accidentally eliminating the correct answer
- Selecting an answer based on an impression

We'll look at the first one here, and the second one in the next section.

To avoid accidentally eliminating the correct answer, we recommend a thought exercise called **the $5 challenge**. In this challenge, you only eliminate an answer choice from contention if you are willing to bet $5 on it being wrong. Why $5? Five dollars is a small but not insignificant amount of money. It's an amount you could afford to lose but wouldn't want to throw away. And while losing $5 once might not hurt too much, doing it twenty times will set you back $100. In the same way, each small decision you make—eliminating a choice here, guessing on a question there—won't by itself impact your score very much, but when you put them all together, they can make a big difference. By holding each answer choice elimination decision to a higher standard, you can reduce the risk of accidentally eliminating the correct answer.

The $5 challenge can also be applied in a positive sense: If you are willing to bet $5 that an answer choice *is* correct, go ahead and mark it as correct.

Summary: Only eliminate an answer choice if you are willing to bet $5 that it is wrong.

Which Answer to Choose

You're taking the test. You've run into a hard question and decided you'll have to guess. You've eliminated all the answer choices you're willing to bet $5 on. Now you have to pick an answer. Why do we even need to talk about this? Why can't you just pick whichever one you feel like when the time comes?

The answer to these questions is that if you don't come into the test with a plan, you'll rely on your impression to select an answer choice, and if you do that, you risk falling into a trap. The test writers know that everyone who takes their test will be guessing on some of the questions, so they intentionally write wrong answer choices to seem plausible. You still have to pick an answer though, and if the wrong answer choices are designed to look right, how can you ever be sure that you're not falling for their trap? The best solution we've found to this dilemma is to take the decision out of your hands entirely. Here is the process we recommend:

Once you've eliminated any choices that you are confident (willing to bet $5) are wrong, select the first remaining choice as your answer.

Whether you choose to select the first remaining choice, the second, or the last, the important thing is that you use some preselected standard. Using this approach guarantees that you will not be enticed into selecting an answer choice that looks right, because you are not basing your decision on how the answer choices look.

This is not meant to make you question your knowledge. Instead, it is to help you recognize the difference between your knowledge and your impressions. There's a huge difference between thinking an answer is right because of what you know, and thinking an answer is right because it looks or sounds like it should be right.

Summary: To ensure that your selection is appropriately random, make a predetermined selection from among all answer choices you have not eliminated.

Test-Taking Strategies

This section contains a list of test-taking strategies that you may find helpful as you work through the test. By taking what you know and applying logical thought, you can maximize your chances of answering any question correctly!

It is very important to realize that every question is different and every person is different: no single strategy will work on every question, and no single strategy will work for every person. That's why we've included all of them here, so you can try them out and determine which ones work best for different types of questions and which ones work best for you.

Question Strategies

Read Carefully

Read the question and answer choices carefully. Don't miss the question because you misread the terms. You have plenty of time to read each question thoroughly and make sure you understand what is being asked. Yet a happy medium must be attained, so don't waste too much time. You must read carefully, but efficiently.

Contextual Clues

Look for contextual clues. If the question includes a word you are not familiar with, look at the immediate context for some indication of what the word might mean. Contextual clues can often give you all the information you need to decipher the meaning of an unfamiliar word. Even if you can't determine the meaning, you may be able to narrow down the possibilities enough to make a solid guess at the answer to the question.

Prefixes

If you're having trouble with a word in the question or answer choices, try dissecting it. Take advantage of every clue that the word might include. Prefixes and suffixes can be a huge help. Usually they allow you to determine a basic meaning. Pre- means before, post- means after, pro - is positive, de- is negative. From prefixes and suffixes, you can get an idea of the general meaning of the word and try to put it into context.

Hedge Words

Watch out for critical hedge words, such as *likely, may, can, sometimes, often, almost, mostly, usually, generally, rarely,* and *sometimes.* Question writers insert these hedge phrases to cover every possibility. Often an answer choice will be wrong simply because it leaves no room for exception. Be on guard for answer choices that have definitive words such as *exactly* and *always.*

Switchback Words

Stay alert for *switchbacks.* These are the words and phrases frequently used to alert you to shifts in thought. The most common switchback words are *but, although,* and *however.* Others include *nevertheless, on the other hand, even though, while, in spite of, despite, regardless of.* Switchback words are important to catch because they can change the direction of the question or an answer choice.

Face Value

When in doubt, use common sense. Accept the situation in the problem at face value. Don't read too much into it. These problems will not require you to make wild assumptions. If you have to go beyond creativity and warp time or space in order to have an answer choice fit the question, then you should move on and consider the other answer choices. These are normal problems rooted in reality. The applicable relationship or explanation may not be readily apparent, but it is there for you to figure out. Use your common sense to interpret anything that isn't clear.

Answer Choice Strategies

Answer Selection

The most thorough way to pick an answer choice is to identify and eliminate wrong answers until only one is left, then confirm it is the correct answer. Sometimes an answer choice may immediately seem right, but be careful. The test writers will usually put more than one reasonable answer choice on each question, so take a second to read all of them and make sure that the other choices are not equally obvious. As long as you have time left, it is better to read every answer choice than to pick the first one that looks right without checking the others.

Answer Choice Families

An answer choice family consists of two (in rare cases, three) answer choices that are very similar in construction and cannot all be true at the same time. If you see two answer choices that are direct opposites or parallels, one of them is usually the correct answer. For instance, if one answer choice says that quantity *x* increases and another either says that quantity *x* decreases (opposite) or says that quantity *y* increases (parallel), then those answer choices would fall into the same family. An answer choice that doesn't match the construction of the answer choice family is more likely to be incorrect. Most questions will not have answer choice families, but when they do appear, you should be prepared to recognize them.

Eliminate Answers

Eliminate answer choices as soon as you realize they are wrong, but make sure you consider all possibilities. If you are eliminating answer choices and realize that the last one you are left with is also wrong, don't panic. Start over and consider each choice again. There may be something you missed the first time that you will realize on the second pass.

Avoid Fact Traps

Don't be distracted by an answer choice that is factually true but doesn't answer the question. You are looking for the choice that answers the question. Stay focused on what the question is asking for so you don't accidentally pick an answer that is true but incorrect. Always go back to the question and make sure the answer choice you've selected actually answers the question and is not merely a true statement.

Extreme Statements

In general, you should avoid answers that put forth extreme actions as standard practice or proclaim controversial ideas as established fact. An answer choice that states the "process should be used in certain situations, if…" is much more likely to be correct than one that states the "process should be discontinued completely." The first is a calm rational statement and doesn't even make a definitive, uncompromising stance, using a hedge word *if* to provide wiggle room, whereas the second choice is a radical idea and far more extreme.

Benchmark

As you read through the answer choices and you come across one that seems to answer the question well, mentally select that answer choice. This is not your final answer, but it's the one that will help you evaluate the other answer choices. The one that you selected is your benchmark or standard for judging each of the other answer choices. Every other answer choice must be compared to your benchmark. That choice is correct until proven otherwise by another answer choice beating it. If you find a better answer, then that one becomes your new benchmark. Once you've decided that no other choice answers the question as well as your benchmark, you have your final answer.

Predict the Answer

Before you even start looking at the answer choices, it is often best to try to predict the answer. When you come up with the answer on your own, it is easier to avoid distractions and traps because you will know exactly what to look for. The right answer choice is unlikely to be word-for-word what you came up with, but it should be a close match. Even if you are confident that you have the right answer, you should still take the time to read each option before moving on.

General Strategies

Tough Questions

If you are stumped on a problem or it appears too hard or too difficult, don't waste time. Move on! Remember though, if you can quickly check for obviously incorrect answer choices, your chances of guessing correctly are greatly improved. Before you completely give up, at least try to knock out a couple of possible answers. Eliminate what you can and then guess at the remaining answer choices before moving on.

Check Your Work

Since you will probably not know every term listed and the answer to every question, it is important that you get credit for the ones that you do know. Don't miss any questions through careless mistakes. If at all possible, try to take a second to look back over your answer selection and make sure you've selected the correct answer choice and haven't made a costly careless mistake (such as marking an answer choice that you didn't mean to mark). This quick double check should more than pay for itself in caught mistakes for the time it costs.

Pace Yourself

It's easy to be overwhelmed when you're looking at a page full of questions; your mind is confused and full of random thoughts, and the clock is ticking down faster than you would like. Calm down and maintain the pace that you have set for yourself. Especially as you get down to the last few minutes of the test, don't let the small numbers on the clock make you panic. As long as you are on track by monitoring your pace, you are guaranteed to have time for each question.

Don't Rush

It is very easy to make errors when you are in a hurry. Maintaining a fast pace in answering questions is pointless if it makes you miss questions that you would have gotten right otherwise. Test writers like to include distracting information and wrong answers that seem right. Taking a little extra time to avoid careless mistakes can make all the difference in your test score. Find a pace that allows you to be confident in the answers that you select.

KEEP MOVING

Panicking will not help you pass the test, so do your best to stay calm and keep moving. Taking deep breaths and going through the answer elimination steps you practiced can help to break through a stress barrier and keep your pace.

Final Notes

The combination of a solid foundation of content knowledge and the confidence that comes from practicing your plan for applying that knowledge is the key to maximizing your performance on test day. As your foundation of content knowledge is built up and strengthened, you'll find that the strategies included in this chapter become more and more effective in helping you quickly sift through the distractions and traps of the test to isolate the correct answer.

Now it's time to move on to the test content chapters of this book, but be sure to keep your goal in mind. As you read, think about how you will be able to apply this information on the test. If you've already seen sample questions for the test and you have an idea of the question format and style, try to come up with questions of your own that you can answer based on what you're reading. This will give you valuable practice applying your knowledge in the same ways you can expect to on test day.

Good luck and good studying!

Principles of Dietetics

Food Science and Nutrient Composition of Foods

Physical and Chemical Properties of Food

Water

Water is composed of two hydrogen atoms connected by one oxygen atom. Water is a liquid at room temperature, but at 32°F (0°C) it becomes a solid. At 212°F (100°C) water boils (at sea level), turning into steam. Atmospheric pressures have an effect on the boiling point of water; the higher the elevation, the lower the atmospheric pressure and, therefore, the lower the boiling point. The freezing point of water can be decreased by the addition of salt, sugar, or alcohol. This is why salt is often used to treat icy roadways in the winter.

Vegetables and Fruits

Composition of Fruits and Vegetables

Cellulose (an insoluble fiber) is an important building component of fruits and vegetables, adding to structural integrity. Hemicelluloses also play a role in structure as do pectic substances. Heating cellulose softens the characteristically rough texture; this may be desirable when eating some vegetables. Fruits and vegetables generally have very high water content. Vegetables have more cellulose than fruit, and water within the cells gives vegetables their crisp texture (turgidity) as exhibited in celery.

Ripening Process

Some fruits may be harvested when ripe, whereas other fruits continue to ripen after they are picked. Bananas are an example of a fruit that continues to ripen after harvest, whereas strawberries do not continue to ripen. Enzymes such as ethylene gas affect ripening, and eventually quality and taste of the fruit will also be affected due to enzymatic action. Ripening affects the sweetness of fruits as starch is converted to sugar. The structural integrity will also change; as enzymes alter the cells, the fruit becomes softer. Generally, refrigeration can slow the degradation process.

Pigments Present

Chlorophyll is the pigment that gives vegetables and fruits their green coloring. Prior to ripening, fruits will often have a green coloring; this is from chlorophyll. As the fruit ripens, the green color will be replaced by other colors because the amount of chlorophyll is decreasing. A strawberry is a good example of a fruit that changes from a greenish color to a bright red when it is fully ripe. Chlorophyll is also affected by heating; when a vegetable is cooked, it may turn a brownish green color. Green beans are a good example of this process taking place; fresh green beans are a brighter green, and upon cooking the color change is evident. Blanching and freezing generally maintain the bright green coloring, making the vegetable more appealing. Carotenoids are responsible for giving fruits and vegetables their yellow and orange coloring, such as in carrots. Red, purple, and blue hues come from the anthocyanins, as seen in blueberries and raspberries. High pH levels will alter the color of anthocyanins, turning them a blue shade, and more acidic mediums turn anthocyanins red.

SUGARS

PHYSICAL AND CHEMICAL PROPERTIES OF SUGARS

There are many different types of sugars, and the sweetness of the sugar depends on the chemical structure as well as temperature. Simple sugars are carbohydrates, and may be monosaccharides or disaccharides, but most sugars encountered are disaccharides. Disaccharides are a combination of monosaccharides. The monosaccharides fructose and glucose can join together to form sucrose, a disaccharide. Sugar not only provides taste to food products, but it also contributes to the appearance and texture of foods. Fructose is the sweetest of sugars, followed by sucrose then glucose. Sugar is water soluble, but the degree of solubility varies depending on the sugar; fructose is most soluble and lactose least soluble in water. The degree of water solubility will have an effect on food product texture.

CARAMELIZATION AND THE MAILLARD REACTION

Caramelization occurs when sugars are heated to high temperatures, resulting in a crispy browning of the product. This often results in desirable product taste and appearance. A good example of the caramelization reaction is exhibited in the heating/torching of crème brûlée. Desserts are not the only products that can be caramelized because sugar is present or can be added to many food types. Onions can be caramelized because they naturally contain sugar.

The Maillard reaction is a browning that occurs when sugar and amino acids are combined primarily through heating, but browning can also occur when this mixture is stored for long periods of time. This reaction results in an attractive product appearance and different taste. The Maillard reaction does not involve enzymes. Oven-roasted meats will brown as they are cooked; this is an example of a Maillard reaction.

FLOUR AND CEREALS

FLOUR CHARACTERISTICS

Whole-wheat flour has undergone less processing, and the grain remains mostly intact; a large portion of the bran and shorts remain. Flour can be refined, which removes much of the bran and shorts; this also results in a white appearance. All-purpose flour is commonly used in baking and is a mixture of hard and soft wheats. All-purpose flour has a relatively high protein content as compared to cake and pastry flours. The protein content of flour dictates the texture of the final product. Pastry and cake flours have less protein content, resulting in softer or flakier products. Bread flour has a higher protein content than all-purpose flour, and this gives bread its heavier and rougher characteristic texture. Using the wrong type of flour can yield an unsatisfactory result.

ROLE OF GLUTEN IN FOOD PRODUCTS

Gluten is a protein found in types of grains including wheat, barley, and rye. Gluten contributes to the characteristics of breads and doughs and is comprised of gliadin and glutenin. Gluten is formed when these two molecules become intertwined. These two components of gluten contribute to bread's ability to rise and to the elasticity of dough. When considering elasticity, pizza dough is a good example of this characteristic. Gluten formation can be slowed with the addition of sugars and fats, whereas a rise in temperature aids gluten development.

MILK AND DAIRY PRODUCTS

FAT, PROTEIN, AND CARBOHYDRATE MAKEUP OF MILK AND DAIRY PRODUCTS

Whole cow's milk is the highest in fat content and contains approximately 3.3% to 3.7% fat. Two percent milk contains approximately 2% fat, low-fat milk contains about 1% fat, and skim milk is very low in fat, with less than 0.5% fat. The content of other nutrients does not vary based on fat content; in general milk is composed of 5% carbohydrates and 3.5 % protein. Lactose is the main carbohydrate present in milk, whereas casein and whey are the primary proteins. The major composition of milk is water.

Pasteurization and Homogenization

Pasteurization of milk products is used to eliminate pathogens and make milk safe to drink. High-temperature, short-time pasteurization is commonly used; milk products are heated to 161°F for 15 seconds to kill dangerous microbes. Unpasteurized milk can be contaminated with E. coli, listeria, and salmonella. Pasteurization does not significantly affect the nutrition content of milk products. Consuming unpasteurized or "raw" milk products does not have any appreciable health benefits and is not advised due to the potential for food-borne illness.

Homogenization results in the physical separation of the fat from the liquid in milk. Through a pressure apparatus, fats are made smaller, and they no longer clump. Although this process is not absolutely necessary, it does make the milk more pleasant to drink. Without homogenization, fat will cluster rather than being uniformly dispersed throughout the milk. The clustering of fat particles will lead to lumpy product, which is typically less appealing to consumers.

Eggs

Physical and Chemical Properties of Eggs

Eggs have a porous outer shell that is made up of calcium. Inside the shell, the vitelline membrane surrounds the yolk. The egg white, known as albumin, provides additional protection for the delicate yolk. Both the yolk and white are high in protein, but the white contains very little fat compared to the yolk. Cholesterol is found within the yolk but not in the egg whites. One large egg contains approximately 70 calories and includes 5 grams of fat, 1.5 grams of saturated fat, and 6 grams of protein. A concern with eggs is the potential presence of salmonella. There is a chance for eggs to contain salmonella, so care must be taken to properly cook eggs to destroy any harmful bacteria.

Egg Quality and Grading

Eggs are graded based on quality, and candling is used to observe specific characteristics. Grade AA is the highest quality, consisting of a normal-appearing outer shell and a firm-looking yolk. Grade A quality eggs show a normal-looking shell, a firm yolk, and some thinning white. Grade A eggs are what you typically buy from the grocery store. Grade B quality eggs may show minor shell defects and a flatter yolk with runny whites. Because of these characteristics, grade B eggs are frequently used by food manufactures to produce egg products. Although eggs have a rather long shelf life when refrigerated, changes do occur with time, affecting the quality of the egg. As moisture and carbon dioxide are lost, the albumin experiences an increase in pH; this change in pH can affect both the taste and appearance of the egg.

Meats, Fish, Poultry, and Meat Alternatives

Structural Components of Meats

Muscle is a component of living creatures; in addition to water, muscle is comprised of proteins called myofibrillar proteins and a smaller amount of fat. Collagen is a tough connective tissue present in abundance in many animals. Heat does act upon collagen to soften the tissue, whereas elastin, another connective tissue, is not affected by heat. The more connective tissue present in meat, the less tender the cut of meat. Fat is another major component of meats; the amount and types of fat vary depending on the animal. Poultry tends to be leaner with less saturated fat than beef products. Many fish such as salmon contain ample amounts of omega-3 fats, which are generally regarded as healthy. Beef products that show fat marbling are often considered to be the most tender and tasty cuts of beef.

Effect of Pigments on Beef Coloring

The red coloring in beef is due to myoglobin, and in the presence of oxygen, myoglobin forms oxymyoglobin, and the result is a bright red color. Further oxidation will result in a brownish gray appearance of meat. Cooking meats has a similar effect upon the color. The myoglobin is converted to oxymyoglobin, and the browning process occurs as the meat cooks. A well-done steak will have a gray-brown appearance, and a rare steak will maintain more a red coloring.

Moist Heat Cooking vs. Dry Heat Cooking

Moist heat cooking utilizes moisture to help prevent the toughening of the meat while providing an ample timeframe for collagen to be broken down and softened. Moist heat is especially advantageous when cooking tough cuts of meat with a lot of connective tissue. Stews are an example of moist heat cooking. When cooking beef stew, chuck roast, which comes from the shoulder, is typically used. Chuck has a lot of connective tissue, which is slowly broken down during the heating process. Other types of moist heating methods include steaming and braising.

Dry heat cooking does not utilize moisture and is best suited for tender cuts of meat. Sirloin can be successfully cooked using dry heat as can poultry and fish. Tender cuts of meat have less collagen and generally do not benefit from prolonged cooking periods. Oven roasting, grilling, and broiling are examples of dry heat cooking.

Fats and Oils

Composition and Structure of Fats

Different types of fats will have varying chemical structures but in fats are composed of carbon, hydrogen, and oxygen. The chemical structure of the fat influences the melting point. Longer chain fats have higher melting points versus short-chain fatty acids. Saturation refers to the amount of "free" space available for hydrogen. Saturated fats are saturated with hydrogen, meaning they cannot hold any more. Unsaturated fats essentially have "free spaces" and do not contain all the hydrogens the chemical structure will allow. Saturated fats tend to be solid at room temperature and have higher melting points. Fats are configured in either a cis or trans formation. Cis formations have the hydrogen atoms on the same side of the double-bonded carbons. Trans formations have the hydrogen atoms diagonally on opposite sides of the double bond. Trans formations have higher melting points than cis formations.

Fat Hydrogenation

Hydrogenation is a chemical process used by the food industry to modify the original structure of fats to achieve a desired product. Hydrogenated oils were frequently found in margarines and commercial baked goods. Hydrogenation increases the melting point, makes the fat more saturated, and increases the shelf life of the fats. In addition, the configuration of the molecule changes to include more trans formations rather than cis formations. Hydrogenation has been shown to have negative impacts on cardiovascular health and is linked to increased levels of low-density lipoprotein (LDL) cholesterol. In 2015, the Food and Drug Administration (FDA) announced that partially hydrogenated oils are not generally recognized as safe and instructed food manufactures to begin removing such oils from products.

Rancid Fats

When fats become rancid, they essentially "go bad" due to chemical changes; rancidity results in an altered taste and appearance. Like most organic compounds, degradation and breakdown begins to affect the chemical structure of fats and result in poor quality. Because of their chemical structure, unsaturated fats degrade more quickly. Because they are not completely saturated with hydrogen atoms and have "free space" available, this configuration attracts oxygen atoms, resulting in oxidation. Regardless of the configuration, all fats are subject to the oxidative process over time. Both light and heat facilitate the oxidative process. Storage of the fat or oil is important; containers that are darker in color may shade the oil from light, and storage in a cool and dark environment will also extend the shelf life. Food manufactures may add antioxidants to oils to help prohibit oxidation; butylated hydroxy anisole (BHA) and butylated hydroxytoluene (BHT) are two common additives.

Leavening Agents

Role of Leavening Agents in Baking

Leavening agents cause breads to rise. Steam is one such leavening agent; steam is created when water reaches the boiling point. Steam causes batter and dough to expand. Carbon dioxide also causes expansion of doughs and batters. Yeast is often used in breads because yeast yields carbon dioxide, thus creating a leavening effect. The addition of acids when combined with alkaline ingredients can also produce a leavening effect through carbon dioxide production. Acidic products include buttermilk and sour cream, whereas baking soda is an alkaline ingredient. Eggs also produce leavening when beaten by trapping air in the batter; this trapped air allows for expansion when the product is baked.

Batters and Doughs

Mixing Methods of Quick Breads

Quick breads do not utilize yeast for leavening; yeast often takes time to rise, whereas other types of leavening agents produce this effect more quickly. In essence, quick breads may be prepared more quickly than yeast breads. Muffins, pancakes, and biscuits are all examples of quick breads. Depending on the product being made, the process and ingredients for producing quick breads differ. In general, a liquid, flour, and sometimes salt are components. The approach to mixing the ingredients varies by product. The biscuit method cuts fat into the dry ingredients, followed by the addition of liquid. The muffin method mixes dry ingredients and liquid ingredients separately at first then combines the two. The conventional method of mixing initially combines the fat and sugar followed by adding egg. Then, dry ingredients are incorporated, followed by the addition of liquids.

Beverages

Coffee

Coffee comes from a plant; the Coffea Arabica and Coffea Robusta are the plants responsible for providing coffee beans. After the beans are harvested and dried, they are roasted to provide optimal flavor. Tannins are naturally present in coffee and contribute to the characteristic bitter taste. Coffee naturally contains caffeine, but it also contains other antioxidants that may contribute to health.

There are variety of ways to brew coffee; the most commonly used method in the United States is the drip method. Most households have a coffeemaker that employs this method. Coffee grounds are put into the machine, and hot water runs over the coffee grounds; typically, the grounds are filtered with a removable paper filter. Coffee percolators are not as commonly used but were once very popular. Percolation involves very hot water continuously passing over the coffee grounds; this method can produce a more bitter-tasting coffee. Single-serve coffee brew machines have become quite popular in recent years. A single pod is place into the machine, and hot water runs through the coffee rounds in the pod. The single-serve method is very quick, but taste may be sacrificed.

Tea

Tea has been around for a very long time, and it is derived from the plant Camellia Sinensis, typically grown in Asia. Like coffee, tea naturally contains caffeine. In general, tea is high in antioxidants; the antioxidant catechin may contribute to the health benefits often associated with tea. Tea types include black tea, green tea, and oolong tea. Tea is derived from the same plant; the process is what determines the type of tea or the final product. All tea is allowed to oxidize, which affects flavor and appearance. Oolong tea is partially oxidized, green tea undergoes very little oxidation, and black tea is allowed to completely oxidize.

Alcoholic Beverages

Alcoholic beverages are generally subdivided into liquor, beer, and wine; each is distinctive in characteristics. Liquor is fermented and distilled; the process of distilling produces a higher alcohol content. Liquors contain the most alcohol by volume; 1.5 ounces is typically 80 proof or 40% alcohol. Beer is produced from a variety of grains; barley is typically used, but wheat, rye, and even corn are sometimes used. Beer alcohol content can vary, but 5% is typical of a 12-oz. beer. Wine is a product of fermented grape juice; the process for making red wine and white wines varies slightly. Ultimately, the type of wine produced will depend on the type or types of grape used in the process. The flavor of wine is dependent on grape type, the amount of aging, and the type of container in which the wine is aged (e.g., an oak barrel).

Functional Foods

There is not an official definition for the term functional food, but functional foods can be considered foods that provide a health benefit beyond basic nourishment of the body. The Academy of Nutrition and Dietetics defines functional foods as "whole foods along with fortified, enriched, or enhanced foods that have a potentially beneficial effect on health when consumed as part of a varied diet on a regular basis at effective levels based on significant standards of evidence." A good example of a true functional food is salmon; salmon is recognized as having heart-healthy effects due to the presence of omega-3 fatty acids. Foods that contain plant sterols are another example of functional foods. Plant sterols may be added to products such as margarine and may have a positive effect upon cholesterol levels. Functional foods do exist and incorporating these foods into the diet may offer health benefits, but it is important to understand that marketing of some "functional foods" is also aimed at selling a product. Investigating the product and ingredients is a wise endeavor for the consumer.

Sensory Evaluation of Food

Using Sensory Evaluation of Food

Sensory evaluation is a scientific approach used by food producers to test and evaluate food products. These tests are carried out by food scientists utilizing a panel of judges to evaluate products using their senses. Such experiments are carried out to produce product formulations that have the potential to be successful in the marketplace. Most people are concerned with how their product tastes; we are unlikely to purchase a product if the taste is unsatisfactory. Food scientists want to know if the food is sweet, salty, bitter, or sour. Does the food leave an aftertaste? Another important factor to consider is visual appeal. If you have ever eaten food that tastes good but looks unappealing, you know this measurement is important for food producers to consider. Color and shape are important considerations. A cake that is generally expected to be fluffy would be a disappointment if it is flat in appearance. Mouthfeel is also an important consideration; is the texture pleasing and expected, or is it hard and lumpy. The smell of the food is also measured; a good smell is a very attractive feature for foods, whereas an off smell can be unappetizing.

Tests Used to Conduct Sensory Evaluations of Food

Single Sample: As the name implies, a single sample is tested to determine whether it is adequate. This type of test may serve as an initial step to determine if product development should continue.

Duo-Trio: This test uses a control and two samples. The objective is to decide which samples differ from the control.

Triangle Test: Three samples are used; two of the samples are the same, whereas a third is unlike the others. The judge must identify the sample that is different.

Descriptive Testing: A scorecard composed of very descriptive sensory words that may be used by the judges to provide additional feedback about the food product.

Hedonic Scale: This is a scale measuring the degree of acceptability; wording will vary, but as an example, the scale may indicate a rating of 1 is "extremely tasty" and a rating of 10 might be "terrible."

Food Preservation

Freezing Foods

Food is subject to spoilage, and a continuous supply of fresh foods is not always available; thus, food preservation is an important component of an adequate supply of food. Freezing can kill or slow the growth of microorganisms that are harmful. Enzymes will not be destroyed by freezing, which means degradation can continue. To stop the enzymatic process, blanching of vegetables is done, and this action also maintains the green coloring in vegetables (due to chlorophyll). Fruits are not suitable for blanching because they are more delicate; ascorbic acid or sugar can help prevent the natural enzymatic process.

Air blast freezing is a very quick method of freezing that employs a blast of very cold

(-30°C to -45°C or -31°F to -49°F), circulating air.

Indirect contact freezing is conducted by cold temperature transfer in which food is placed on a flat holding plate, and the shelves holding the food contain frigid liquids.

Immersion freezing involves immersing or submerging the food into a very cold liquid such as sodium chloride; the liquid can also be a cryogenic liquid such as are nitrogen and carbon dioxide.

Canning Foods

Canning of foods may take place on a large commercial scale or may take place in the home. The goal is essentially the same—to achieve a safe, highly shelf-stable product. Canned products can be held for approximately 2 years and still maintain their safety; nutrient loss will occur during this time.

Heat is the key to canning; the presence of heat combined with adequate time and correct temperatures are all factors in safe canning. A major pathogen concern among canned products is Clostridium botulinum; this pathogen produces spores that are very heat resistant. Foods that are low in acid, such as most vegetables, should be canned under pressurization to reduce the risk of botulinum contamination. Fruits may be canned using a water bath method. Fruits are placed in glass jars and immersed in boiling water. Because fruits are generally higher in acid content (lower pH), pressurization is not necessary.

Beyond the initial destruction of pathogenic organisms, it is critical that cans and jars are sealed properly. An inadequate seal allows oxygen to enter and opens the door for spoilage.

FOOD DEHYDRATION

Food dehydration significantly reduces the moisture content from foods, thus making them more shelf stable and less subject to deterioration or contamination. Because most microbes require moisture, drying foods destroys bacteria, yeast, and mold, and airtight packaging helps maintain the preservation and retard growth. Commercial means of dehydration include spray drying, freeze drying, and vacuum belt drying. Many types of foods can be dehydrated including meats (beef jerky), fruits (grapes and bananas,) and even vegetables (green beans). Physical and nutrient changes occur during the dehydration process. The removal of water content will have an obvious effect on the product's appearance. The product may appear shrunken or shriveled due to the loss of water (water adds to plumpness and shape). Color changes may also be evident as browning tends to occur because of the Maillard reaction. Dehydration also causes protein denaturation and vitamin C loss.

ADDITIONAL PRESERVATION METHODS

Sugar provides a hospitable medium for food preservation by means of osmosis, which limits the water available for microbes to grow. Jellies and jams are effectively preserved, and microbes are killed with addition of sugar and boiling heat.

Freeze-drying is actually a form of food dehydration. As opposed to traditional dehydration methods, with freeze-drying, foods are first frozen, and then water is extracted. Freeze-drying produces a more visually appealing product because the original size of the food is better maintained as opposed to a shrunken appearance.

Food irradiation uses gamma rays to kill microorganisms and is an effective means of preserving food while maintaining food integrity. According to the Food and Drug Administration (FDA), irradiating foods is a safe process, and nutritional quality is not comprised by this form of food preservation.

FOOD PROCESSING

PROCESSED FOOD

Processed foods encompass a broad range of foods. Strictly speaking, processed foods are foods that have been changed in some way prior to delivery to the customer. This certainly includes many foods, and a processed food is not always synonymous with unhealthy. Gone are the days where most people go to their gardens to pick fresh foods and have farm animals to utilize for protein sources. Although this way of life certainly still exists, we live in a society in which food is transported from one region of the country to another. Although fresh fruits are transported and distributed across state lines or country borders, we also rely on the convenience of processed foods to safely fill our dinner tables and lunch boxes. Processed foods are more shelf stable so they can be kept for longer periods of time either with or without refrigeration or freezing. Food processing may involve canning, drying, and other forms of food preservation such as smoking and salting. Milling of grains is another type of food processing that turns grains into more usable forms. Pasteurization of milk, egg products, and juices take place to ensure a safer product. Food preservation provides us the opportunity to safely enjoy fruits and vegetables in December even when they are not in season. Without food processing, many conveniences and healthy options would not be available.

Food Additives

The addition of food additives is an example of food processing. According to the Food and Drug Administration (FDA), a food additive can be "any substance added to food." The FDA cites the legal definition of a food additive as "any substance the intended use of which results or may reasonably be expected to result, directly or indirectly, in it becoming a component or otherwise affecting the characteristics of any food." Food additives that are generally recognized as safe do not need prior approval before inclusion in a food product. There are many types of additives, and they are used for multiple purposes. For example, salt may be added to foods for the purpose of preservation and/or taste enhancement. Folic acid and vitamin D may be added to food products to provide nutritive value. Dyes may be used to improve color, and citric acid may be used to control pH. Cornstarch and dextrin provide texture for foods, whereas yeasts and baking powder are used for leavening.

Safety of Food Additives

Many of the additives used in foods are the same ingredients we use at home in our own kitchens. According to the Food and Drug Administration (FDA), food additives are used in food to maintain or improve safety or freshness, improve or maintain nutrition, and improve texture, taste, and appearance. The FDA maintains a database of additives used in foods, and food additives are regulated. Still, concerns about additive safety are abundant, but the FDA does take measures that promote safety, and their actions are based upon prevailing, available scientific evidence. The FDA is tasked with evaluating food additives and considers four main factors: composition and properties, the amount one would typically consume, health effects, and other safety factors. If an additive is ultimately approved, the FDA may set limits on how the additive can be used. Beyond initial approval, the FDA monitors new additives and reserves the right to re-review and revoke approval. Other food additives known as generally recognized as safe (GRAS) are not subject to approval. Based on long-standing use and scientific evidence, these ingredients are accepted to be safe. Examples of such ingredients include: sugar, salt, and spices. Although there cannot be a 100% guarantee of safety with food additives, the processes in place aim to provide a safe food supply for all Americans.

Food Packaging

Food is commercially packaged to maintain safety and quality and to provide a means for storage and easy transport. Glass jars are frequently used to package products such as spaghetti sauce, pickles, and other sauces. Glass may be clear, offering the consumer an opportunity to view the product, or it may be colored to prevent light penetration, thus helping to prevent degradation. Glass does not impart a taste to the product, which may occur with metal containers. Metal containers are widely used, and you may see drinks, vegetables, soups, cream, and other products packaged in metal cans consisting of aluminum or steel. Metal containers are lightweight and relatively durable compared to glass. Plastics are another type of package commonly used in the food industry in part because they are cost-effective. Plastics or polymers are used to house an almost endless variety of products including milk, oils, cheeses, frozen microwave meals, and margarines. Bisphenol-A (BPA) is a component of some plastics. Although the Food and Drug Administration (FDA) has deemed it safe for current use, BPA is no longer used in the production of infant baby bottles, sippy cups, or infant formula. Other food manufactures have voluntarily chosen to eliminate BPA from their packaging. Paper and paperboard may also be used to package products such as milk, snack foods, cereals, and pastas.

Food Biotechnology and Genetic Engineering

Food biotechnology is also referred to as genetic engineering and involves genetically modifying a food to produce a desired outcome. This type of modification is unlike forms of food processing.

According to the Food and Drug Administration (FDA), the majority of genetically modified foods are corn, cotton, canola, and soybean. Genetically modified foods may be engineered to resist insects and disease. This should result in fewer pesticides being used and a greater crop yield, which is beneficial from health and economic standpoints. In addition, foods can be modified to withstand environmental barriers to successful crop growing. For instance, drought conditions and cold climates can adversely affect many types of plants; these disadvantages can be overcome through food biotechnology. Foods can even be modified to exhibit certain nutrition enhancements, such as increasing beta-carotene or iron. Like other foods, genetically modified foods are regulated by the FDA, and steps are taken to ensure safety.

Scientific Basis for Preparation and Storage

Techniques of Food Preparation

Moist Heat Methods of Food Preparation

Braising: First the meat is typically browned in a skillet to lock in the juices; then the meat is transitioned to a moist heat cooking method and cooked in a juice such as broth. Typically, the meat is cooked slowly for a long period of time. Examples of meats that are commonly braised include roasts and short ribs.

Simmering: Liquids are kept very hot but not quite at the boiling point. Many recipes will call for simmering of ingredients. Spaghetti sauce or marinara sauce may be simmered to allow liquids to dissipate and spices to infiltrate the sauce.

Stewing: This involves slowly cooking at high temperatures in juices; beef stew is a good example of this cooking method.

Steaming: Food is cooked from the steam given off by boiling water. Vegetables are commonly steamed.

Boiling: Food is cooked in boiling water; examples include rice and pasta.

Dry Heat Methods of Food Preparation

Frying: Foods are cooked in oil; foods may be deep fried, which involves completely covering the foods with oil (French fries), or smaller but significant amounts may be used for pan frying (fried green tomatoes).

Sautéing: Foods are cooked in a small amount of fat or oil; the food is not covered in oil. Vegetables are commonly sautéed.

Roasting: Roasting is essentially baking, but we often refer to roasting when talking about meats and vegetables; foods can be baked for shorter periods of time, or items may be slow roasted. Many items can be baked, including potatoes, tenderloin, chicken, and vegetables.

Grilling: Foods are cooked via a direct flame from heat below the food. Many items can be successfully grilled, including hamburgers, steaks, and vegetables.

Broiling: Food is cooked in an oven utilizing radiant, high heat emitted from the top of the oven; meats are good candidates for broiling.

Effects of Techniques and Methods on Aesthetic Properties and Nutrient Retention

The method of cooking can have an impact on the final nutrient content of foods. Some methods of cooking preserve nutrients rather well, whereas others tend to destroy or promote nutrient loss.

Many factors such as time and temperature also affect nutrient retention. Vitamin C is not very heat stable, so it is expected that losses of vitamin C will occur in food. Minerals tend to be more heat stable and less affected by cooking compared to many vitamins. Boiling of foods tends to promote the greatest loss of nutrients; water-soluble vitamins may be leeched into the water. Frying will promote some loss of nutrients and deep frying may promote greater losses with higher temperatures and immersion in oil. Sautéing is typically one of the best methods for preserving nutrients. Because foods are cooked quickly in a small amount of oil, losses are minimized. Changes in food appearance also occur with cooking. Caramelization causes browning and produces a crispy texture. Meats will brown when cooking, thus improving their appearance. Foods can also lose water during cooking and therefore lose plumpness or volume. Color losses (chlorophyll) may also occur when foods are heated; broccoli loses its bright green coloring and takes on a more green-brown appearance.

Roles of Food Additives

Antioxidants may be added to food to provide a more stable product by increasing shelf life through limiting the oxidative process. Examples of antioxidants include ascorbic acid and vitamin E.

Emulsifiers are necessary to allow for proper mixing of liquids so that it is appealing and more edible. Mayonnaise is an emulsion; without an emulsifier mayonnaise would be separated into a solid and liquid form. Lecithin and monoglycerides are examples of emulsifiers.

Humectants are used in foods that need to retain moisture. Because moisture can promote microbial growth over time, humectants may be added, which in turn bind to the water; this process extends shelf life. Humectant examples include salt and glycerin.

Stabilizers impact the texture of foods by adding a smoothing quality while preventing separation. Without the use of stabilizers many foods would be lumpy or have an inconsistent texture. Stabilizers used include pectin, gelatin, and hydrolyzed vegetable protein.

Antimicrobial agents work to prevent the growth of microbes such as bacteria or mold. Examples of antimicrobial additives include sodium nitrite and sodium benzoate.

Sources of Data, Labels

2016 Nutrition Facts Food Label

The Food and Drug Administration (FDA) governs food labeling practices. The Nutrition Labeling and Education Act (NLEA) says most foods must have a label, and if health claims are made, additional requirements must be met. In 2016, labeling changes were finalized that included requiring manufactures to list the actual amounts of vitamin D, calcium, iron, and potassium (in addition to the percent daily value). Based on scientific feedback, daily values are also being updated for several nutrients. Specifying "added sugars" in grams is also new. There is no longer a requirement to list vitamin A and vitamin C. The "calories from fat" category is no longer required. The new food label will also reflect a change in serving sizes. According to the FDA, the law indicates serving sizes are to be based on amounts consumers are typically eating rather than what people should be eating. Serving sizes on food labels have generally not reflected reality in that they are too small and will be updated.

% Daily Value

The % daily value listed on the food label is based on a 2,000-calorie diet. If the food label indicates 14% for dietary fiber, the consumer knows one serving of the product he or she is eating provides 14% of his or her daily fiber needs. Of course, not everyone should follow a 2,000-calorie diet.

Because individual needs will vary, the 2,000-calorie reference serves as a guide. The daily values are listed to help consumers make appropriate food choices and are based on the Recommended Dietary Allowances (RDA).

Health Claims

Health claims that are allowed by the Food and Drug Administration (FDA) for food labeling and dietary supplement labeling fall into three categories: health claims, nutrient content claims, and structure and function claims. Health claims indicate a relationship between the food and a health or medical condition. According to the FDA, an example of a health claim is that "adequate calcium throughout life may reduce the risk of osteoporosis." Prior to including a health claim on a food label, permission from the FDA must be obtained. Nutrient content claims indicate how much of a nutrient is contained in the food product. Terminology included in these claims include high, low, or lite. "Low-fat" or "high calcium" are specific examples that could be included on a food label. Structure and function claims relate a nutrient to a bodily function. According to the FDA, a structure or function statement could be: "fiber maintains bowel regularity." Food manufacturers are not required to notify or obtain permission from the FDA to use structure or function claims (dietary supplements are subject to different restrictions).

Macro and Micronutrients Sources

Macronutrients

Macronutrients are carbohydrates, proteins, and fats. The body requires large amounts of these nutrients to function properly. Carbohydrates are the body's primary source of fuel or energy. Carbohydrates provide 4 calories per gram. Of the macronutrients, carbohydrates should compose most of our dietary intake (50%–60% of daily calories for most individuals). Carbohydrates come most from plant sources such as grains, fruits, and starchy vegetables, but dairy products also contain carbohydrates. Protein is involved in muscle composition and serves many other important roles. Like carbohydrates, protein provides 4 calories per gram. Dietary protein sources are mainly from meats, fish, and poultry, but beans, nuts, and dairy also contain protein. Fats are components of cell members and aid in digestion; they can be used as energy when other sources are depleted. Dietary sources of fat typically come from meats, fish, dairy and oils.

Micronutrients

Micronutrients are vitamins and minerals, and compared to macronutrients, the body only requires small amounts of micronutrients. Examples of micronutrients include the fat-soluble vitamins D, E, K, and A, and the water-soluble C and the B vitamins. Also included, but not limited to the micronutrient class, are the minerals calcium, iron, sodium, potassium, and magnesium. Milk and dairy products are prominent sources of both calcium and vitamin D. Vitamin E is commonly found in nuts and oils; vitamin A is concentrated in carrots, sweet potatoes, and other carotenoids; and vitamin K is found in leafy green vegetables. The B vitamins will generally be found in grains and fortified cereals, whereas vitamin C can be found in vegetables and fruits. The best source of iron is meats, but some whole grains and leafy green vegetables also contain iron. Sodium can be found in abundance in a large variety of dietary sources, whereas potatoes and bananas are good sources of potassium. Fish, nuts, and whole grains provide excellent sources of magnesium.

Phytochemicals

Phytochemicals are components of food that are believed to offer protective health benefits. These chemicals occur naturally in plant-based foods, making vegetables, fruits, and whole grains even more attractive. Specific, recommended levels of intake have not been developed for phytochemicals because additional research is still needed to study these chemicals. As dietitians, we can recommend consuming a plant-based diet because doing so is related to better health, and phytochemicals are thought to play a role in the protective effect. There are thousands of phytochemicals found in foods. Some of the better known phytochemicals include flavonoids, anthocyanins, carotenoids, and lignans. Additional studies are needed, but research suggests phytochemicals may play a role in cancer and cardiovascular disease prevention. Studies linking phytochemicals to a decreased risk for type 2 diabetes and neurodegenerative diseases like Parkinson's and Alzheimer's are also promising.

NUTRIENT DATABASES AND NUTRIENT ANALYSIS

Nutrient databases house data on specific nutrients in foods. Although there are commercial databases available to purchase and use, the United States Department of Agriculture (USDA) provides a massive, online database available for anyone to use. The database may be searched by food or by entering a nutrient or combination of nutrients. The output includes information on macronutrients in addition to specific vitamins, minerals, and fiber.

Nutrient databases can be used by dietitians to conduct nutrient analysis of foods. An analysis will help determine approximately the amount of calories, fat, and protein provided by each food item. Additional analysis can be done that includes fiber content, a specific breakdown of fats, or other vitamins and minerals of interest.

Nutrition and Supporting Sciences

Function of Nutrients and Nonnutritive Substances

Function of Carbohydrates Within the Body

Carbohydrates supply the body with energy and are the main source of fuel for humans. The chemicals' structure for carbohydrates consists of carbon, hydrogen, and oxygen. Carbohydrates can be divided into three major subcategories: monosaccharides, oligosaccharides, and polysaccharides. Fructose, galactose, and glucose are examples of monosaccharides, which are considered simple sugars. The class oligosaccharides consist of the maltose, lactose, and sucrose, which are also termed disaccharides. Polysaccharides include glycogen, fiber, and starch; they are often referred to as complex carbohydrates. Glycogen is the stored form of glucose; the capability to convert glucose to glycogen is essential for the body to function efficiently.

Function of Proteins Within the Body

Dietary protein provides energy at 4 kcals/g, but more importantly protein is composed of amino acids, which are essential for life. Complete dietary proteins generally come from animal sources and contain all the amino acids required. In contrast, incomplete dietary proteins do not provide all the necessary amino acids. Incomplete proteins are contained in plant food sources. Proteins contribute to the composition of the human body; most protein is concentrated in muscle, followed by the organs. The role of proteins in the body are vast. Amino acids are involved in the production of several hormones such as tyrosine and insulin. Enzymes are also composed of proteins; enzymes facilitate chemical reactions within the body. Collagen and muscles are also comprised of proteins. Proteins serve as carriers for other substances in the body; albumin is an example.

Function of Fats Within the Body

Fats are also known as lipids, and dietary lipids provide more energy than either carbohydrates or protein at 9 kcals/g. Lipids have many important functions within the human body, including insulation, cell membrane integrity and composition, and hormone structure. Lipids are divided into several different classes according to their structure. Fatty acids have a simple chemical makeup. Fatty acids may be saturated or unsaturated and can be essential or nonessential. Essential fatty acids are a necessary component of the human diet; examples include linoleic and alpha-linolenic acid. If these fatty acids are excluded from the diet, growth failure and cognitive implications ensue. Another classification of fats is sterols and steroids. Cholesterols is a member of this class and has important roles in the development of hormones and vitamin D. Phospholipids deviate from the structure of other lipids in that they contain phosphate. Phospholipids are components of cell membranes and are structurally significant in the myelin sheath of nerve tissues. Another class, glycolipids, function primarily as structural contributors within the body; this includes the composition of brain tissue.

Fat-Soluble Vitamins

The fat soluble vitamins are D, E, K, and A.

Vitamin D: Vitamin D plays an important role in bone mineralization through the uptake and release of calcium and phosphorus, but it is critical in many lesser known functions. Vitamin D is found primarily in fortified foods, but the body is able to synthesize vitamin D when sunlight exposure is sufficient. Calcitriol is the active form of vitamin D and acts as a hormone. Vitamin D is involved in immune function and nutrient absorption—specifically calcium and phosphorus.

Vitamin E: Vitamin E is actually an antioxidant; this role makes vitamin E interesting in the role of disease prevention, but this role as an antioxidant is also important to preserve normal cell function. Vitamin E works to prevent oxidation of cell membranes, thus it is essential in preventing cell damage and deterioration that naturally occurs.

Vitamin K: Vitamin K plays a role in bone mineralization and blood clotting. Although dietary sources exist, the body is able to produce vitamin K in the intestines from the presence of bacteria.

Vitamin A: Vitamin A has a variety of functions within the body—one of the most notable is its significant role in eyesight. For its role in vision, vitamin A is actually metabolized in the retina. Rhodopsin, which is involved in night vision, is made from vitamin A. Vitamin A is also involved in epithelial cell function, growth and bone metabolism and functions as an antioxidant.

Vitamin C and Folic Acid

Vitamin C is also known as ascorbic acid. Vitamin C has several important roles within the body. Among these functions include synthesis of collagen, carnitine (an amino acid involved in energy production), and tyrosine (involved in melanin production and neurotransmitter production). Vitamin C also functions as an antioxidant. As an antioxidant, ascorbic acid is thought to play a role in the prevention of cardiovascular disease, some cancers, and macular degeneration. A deficiency of vitamin C can result in scurvy.

Folic acid or folate is involved in cell division and cell production. Folic acid plays a role in deoxyribonucleic acid (DNA) metabolism and amino acid metabolism. Folate deficiency has been linked to neural tube defects, and deficiency is thought to play a role in the development of some cancers. Normal cell division is adversely affected when the body is deficient in folate; a folate deficiency is known as megaloblastic anemia.

Thiamin, Riboflavin, Niacin, and Pyridoxamine

Thiamin is also known as vitamin B_1. Thiamin functions primarily as a coenzyme and is involved in carbohydrate metabolism and energy production. A deficiency of thiamin is known as beriberi. Specifically, thiamin deficiency as a result of alcoholism is called Wernicke-Korsakoff syndrome.

Riboflavin is known as vitamin B_2 and has a variety of metabolic roles. Deficiency of riboflavin is known as ariboflavinosis; alcoholics are more susceptible to riboflavin deficiency due to poor intake.

Niacin is also known as vitamin B_3. Niacin functions as a coenzyme in many capacities and plays a prominent role in glycolysis and the Krebs cycle. Pellagra is the term for deficiency of niacin.

Pantothenic Acid, Biotin, and Pyridoxamine, and Cobalamin

Pyridoxamine is also referred to as vitamin B_6. Vitamin B_6 functions as an enzyme and coenzyme. Pyridoxamine is involved in hemoglobin synthesis and is involved in metabolism. Those at risk for vitamin B_6 deficiency include alcoholics, the elderly, and renal patients on dialysis.

Pantothenic acid is involved in the formation of coenzyme A, which is essential for nutrient metabolism. Deficiency of pantothenic acid usually does not occur alone—typically there would be other nutrient deficiencies as well.

Biotin also serves as a coenzyme and is involved in metabolism. Deficiency is uncommon but can occur due to malabsorption or alcoholism.

Cobalamin is also referred to as vitamin B_{12}. Cobalamin is involved in the metabolism of folate. A deficiency of cobalamin may result in megaloblastic anemia.

Calcium and Magnesium

Calcium has a variety of functions but is well-known for its contribution to strong teeth and bones. In addition, calcium is involved in the transmission of nerve impulses and cell function and plays a role in muscle contraction. A lack of recommended calcium may result in the disease rickets in children, and a lack of adequate calcium may contribute to osteopenia and osteoporosis in older adults.

Magnesium, like calcium, is essential for strong bones. Magnesium and calcium work together in bone metabolism; magnesium is necessary for parathyroid hormone secretion. Magnesium also plays a role in energy production, the synthesis of deoxyribonucleic acid (DNA) and ribonucleic acid (RNA), heart rhythm, and muscular contractions. A deficiency of magnesium is rare. Susceptible individuals include alcoholics, the elderly, and those with diseases resulting in malabsorption.

Sodium, Chloride, and Potassium

Sodium is important in fluid and electrolyte balance in addition to muscle contraction. Sodium deficiency is rare, and sodium concentrations are well regulated, but sodium losses could result from intense sweating.

Chloride works as an electrolyte in concert with sodium to maintain fluid balance and also composes gastric acids. In the diet, chloride is generally consumed with sodium. Chloride deficiency is not common, but fluid loss from prolonged diarrhea or vomiting could upset the balance.

Potassium, like sodium and chloride, is involved in fluid homeostasis and is also involved in muscle contraction. Potassium is concentrated inside the cells; it is known as an intracellular cation.

Copper, Iron, and Chromium

Copper functions as an enzyme and is involved in energy production, iron metabolism, and collagen synthesis. Copper deficiency is not widespread, but those more susceptible include individuals with malabsorption problems, cystic fibrosis patients, and individuals consuming excess zinc.

Iron composes a major portion of hemoglobin, which is involved in the vital activity of oxygen transport. A deficiency of iron is called iron deficiency anemia, and this is common. The problem is encountered most often in infants and younger children, adolescents, females of childbearing age, and pregnant women. Also, anyone with prolonged loss of blood or absorptive problems, such as those with Celiac disease, may become iron deficient.

Chromium's most important role may be in the action of insulin, but the exact mechanism is not completely understood. Chromium deficiency is quite rare.

Zinc, Manganese, and Fluoride

Zinc is involved in a variety of bodily functions including taste and smell, energy metabolism, and protein synthesis. Zinc deficiency is uncommon, but alcoholics and those receiving total parenteral nutrition without zinc are more likely to be affected.

Manganese is involved in lipid and glucose metabolism as well as collagen and bone growth. Manganese deficiency generally does not occur under normal circumstances, but toxicity can occur in those experiencing liver failure.

Fluoride is known for its role in strengthening tooth enamel. A lack of sufficient fluoride may lead to dental cavities.

Phosphorus, Selenium, and Iodine

Phosphorus contributes to the structural integrity of teeth and bones and is a component of phospholipids. Phosphorus deficiency is rarely observed.

Selenium functions are not well understood, but selenium's most notable role include that of an enzyme cofactor and its role in iodine metabolism. Selenium deficiency is not widespread but can occur with total parenteral nutrition.

Iodine is involved in the synthesis of thyroid hormones. Iodine deficiency can cause severe cognitive deficits; to help curb such problems, iodine has been added to table salt. Iodine deficiency continues to be a problem in many developing countries.

Nutrient, Energy Needs and Feeding Patterns Throughout the Life Span

Nutritional Needs During Pregnancy and Lactation

Pregnancy is unlike any other time in life. Although there is not a necessity for an expectant mother to "eat for two," her intake must increase to support the many changes and growing fetus. Weight gain during pregnancy on average is 25 to 35 lbs. If underweight prior to pregnancy, a greater weight gain of 28 to 40 lbs. is suggested. If overweight prior to conception, 15 to 25 lbs. are optimal.

As expected, additional energy is required during pregnancy. During the first trimester, energy needs are not expected to increase. During the second trimester, an additional 340 kcals/day is warranted, and during the third trimester the daily reference intakes (DRI) for energy is 452 kcals/day.

Protein needs increase during the second part of pregnancy and the recommended daily allowance (RDA) for this time is 1.1 g/kg/day.

During pregnancy (and ideally prior to conception) folic acid supplementation of 400 micrograms is recommended to help prevent neural tube defects and other congenital malformations.

Energy needs during lactation are demanding. Lactation during the first 6 months requires an additional 330 kcals/day, and during the second 6 months postpartum, 400 additional kcals/day is recommended.

Nutritional Needs During Infancy

The rapid growth associated with infancy results in a tremendous amount of energy needed to support the growth changes. Energy needs vary by age, and the estimated energy requirements are calculated using the following equations:

0–3 months: (89 x infant weight (kg) - 100) + 175

4–6 months: (89 x infant weight (kg) - 100) + 56

7–12 months: (89 x infant weight (kg) - 100) + 22

The daily reference intakes (DRI) for protein is as follows:

0–6 months: 1.52 g/kg/d

6–12 months: 1.2 g/kg/d

Infants less than 12 months of age should consume at least 30 grams of fat per day. Of particular emphasis are alpha-linolenic and linoleic acid, which are essential fatty acids. Breast milk naturally contains these fats, and most infant formulas are fortified.

Breast milk or formula is the only requirement for infants during the first 6 months of life, but solid foods are introduced anywhere from 4 to 6 months of age. A slow progression of solid food initiates with the introduction of cereal, followed by pureed vegetables and fruits and finger foods. The infant gradually progresses with different textures and is able to tolerate strained and chopped foods followed by the introduction of table foods at 9 to 12 months of age.

Nutritional Needs of Children

Although the growth rate has slowed since infancy, children are still experiencing rapid growth and development. As children grow, they become more independent, and this includes dietary independence. Many factors influence dietary intake but possibly none more than the family. It is important to set a healthy tone for dietary intake and offer a variety of healthy choices. The prevalence of obesity has risen in recent decades, and to curb this trend early education and intervention are necessary. Children may attend daycare or school; this too influences the eating patterns of this age group along with peers.

Estimated Energy Requirements (EER):

Males and females ages 13 to 35 months: (89 x child's weight [kg] – 100) + 20

Girls 3 to 8 years: 135.3 – (30.8 x age [years]) + plus activity factor x {(10 x weight [kg]) + (934 x height [m])} + 20

Boys 3 – 8 years: 88.5 – (61.9 x age [years]) + physical activity factor x {(26.7 x weight [kg]) + (903 x height [m]} + 20

With age, protein needs decrease. At 1 to 3 years of age, protein needs are 1.05 g/kg/day, whereas at 4 to 8 years of age, protein needs drop to 0.95 g/kg/day.

Nutritional Needs of Adolescents

Adolescence and the teenage years bring with it many changes. Growing independence brings more choices for food beyond the family meal. School and peer influences may have significant impacts on the dietary patterns for this age group. Nevertheless, continued promotion of healthy dietary intake is important. Due the varying growth and changes associated with puberty, actual nutrient needs will vary depending on age and stage of development/growth. The following indicates the estimated energy requirements (EER):

Girls 9 to 18 years: 135.3 – (30.8 x age [years]) + physical activity factor x {(10 x weight [kg]) + (934 x height [m])} + 25

Boys 9 to 18 years: 88.5 – (61.9 x age [years]) + physical activity factor x {(26.7 x weight [kg]) + 903 x height [m])} + 25

The recommended daily allowance (RDA) for protein for the 9- to 13-year-old group is 0.95 g/kg/day, and for 14- to 18-year-olds the requirement decreases to 0.85 g/kg/day.

NUTRITIONAL NEEDS OF ADULTS AND THE AGING POPULATION

During the adult years, the goal is to maintain a healthy diet and a healthy weight. Growth should be complete, so nutrient needs should generally stabilize. As an individual advances in age, a healthy diet continues to be important, but additional needs may arise as a part of the aging process.

Recommended Daily Allowance (RDA) for Protein (Adults): 0.80 g/kg/day

The progression in aging may result in a variety of physical changes. These changes can affect dietary intake and nutrient needs. With aging may come poor eyesight and hearing; poor eyesight can affect the ability to shop for or prepare foods. Taste and smell may also be adversely affected, resulting in poor intake. Mobility issues may result, which can produce a host of problems related to intake. Mental changes may occur that affect the desire to eat. In addition, other health problems including cardiovascular disease and gastrointestinal disease may have adverse effects. These are all issues that must be managed because malnutrition is a concern with the aging population.

Nutrient needs vary greatly in this population because there are so many variables to consider. Energy needs can be estimated using the Mifflin-St. Jeor equation, and protein needs may increase to 1.0 to 1.2 g/kg/day.

HERBALS, BOTANICALS, AND SUPPLEMENTS

According to the Food and Drug Administration (FDA), "The law defines dietary supplements in part as products taken by mouth that contain a 'dietary ingredient.' Dietary ingredients include vitamins, minerals, amino acids, and herbs or botanicals as well as other substances that can be used to supplement the diet." The use of supplements may fall under the terminology complementary or alternative medicine. Many different types of supplements exist, and their intended purposes vary. Botanicals or herbals may be used interchangeably, but they are derived from plants. Examples of herbals and botanicals are garlic, gingko biloba, and St. John's Wart. Other types of supplements include vitamins and minerals. These supplements may be sold as a multivitamin that provides a combination of vitamins and minerals or may be packaged individually. Examples include calcium, vitamin E, and fish oil. It is important for the dietitian to be familiar with supplements to evaluate their use in patients.

GASTROINTESTINAL

INGESTION AND DIGESTION

Food is taken in by mouth (ingested) then is mixed with saliva and chewed. The food is swallowed and travels through the esophagus into the stomach. Digestion truly begins in the stomach due to the breakdown of food from gastric acids and enzymes. When this phase is complete, the contents are referred to as chyme, and the contents pass into the small intestine through the pyloric valve. The small intestine, divided into the duodenum, jejunum, and ileum, is where the majority of digestion takes place. Specifically, the duodenum, the first section of the small intestines, is the site of the most digestion. With the help of enzymes and hormones, food is further broken down, and the majority of nutrients are absorbed. The remaining contents pass through the ileocecal valve into the large intestines. Very few nutrients or fluids are absorbed in the colon. The final portion of the digestive tract is the rectum, and the remaining contents exit the digestive tract through the anus.

ABSORPTION

Digestion is not just a physical process that begins in the mouth, it is also a chemical process facilitated by enzymatic action and hormones. The enzyme salivary lipase is secreted in the mouth, thus initiating the breakdown of starch and fats. In the stomach, pepsin begins the work of breaking down proteins. Gastric lipase contributes to the breakdown of some fats. In the small intestine, bile salts are instrumental in absorption of fat-soluble vitamins and lipids. Pancreatic lipase and colipase are pancreatic enzymes that further aid in the digestion of fats, whereas pancreatic amylase facilitates the digestion of starch. Trypsin and chymotrypsin from the pancreas further break down protein. The small intestine is structurally designed to absorb nutrients. The small intestines consist of many folds and villi; as such the surface area for absorption is massive.

Metabolism

Glycogenesis

Conversion of glucose to glycogen takes place in the liver; glycogen is also stored in the liver and muscles. When the body detects excess glucose in the bloodstream, the process of glycogenesis initiates. Glucose-6-phosphate begins the process of glycogenesis, and insulin facilitates the process. This process is impaired in individuals with type 1 diabetes because of the lack of insulin (insulin stimulates glucose uptake). Through a series of chemical reactions, the excess glucose is converted to glycogen for use as energy at a later time. Because we are not constantly eating and providing a continuous stream of carbohydrates, low circulating levels of glucose in the bloodstream signal the body to access "energy reserves." The process of glycogenesis provides metabolic balance and allows the human body to operate seamlessly.

Glycolysis

Glycolysis involves the breakdown of glucose into either pyruvate or lactate. Glucose breakdown via this pathway is necessary to produce the large amounts of energy that result from the Krebs cycle. The presence or absence of oxygen during the process determines the end product. In aerobic glycolysis, pyruvate is produced. In anaerobic glycolysis, lactate becomes the end product from the conversion of pyruvate. Pyruvate production is significant because it is involved in the Krebs cycle in which it is completely oxidized. Typically, pyruvate becomes the end product, and this is the preferred route that will ultimately result in sufficient energy release. Under conditions where the body is lacking oxygen, such as the case with vigorous exercise, lactate is produced. Less energy is released during the lactic acid cycle as the body is not designed to sustain prolonged periods of oxygen debt.

Krebs Cycle

The Krebs cycle is also referred to as the citric acid cycle. This metabolic pathway causes the release of energy; this pathway is the most critical because it accounts for the majority of energy utilized from foods. Although the process is complex and microscopic, in broad terms, the Krebs cycle could be thought of as extracting energy from the food we eat. This cycle takes place in the mitochondria of cells. The process initiates with the acetyl CoA formed from the breakdown of nutrients such as fatty acids or glucose. Pyruvate enters the cycle as a result of glycolysis.

Steps in Krebs Cycle:

1. Citrate is formed.
2. Citrate is isomerized (molecules are changed into different molecules).
3. Isocitrate dehydrogenase reaction produces energy by reoxidizing NADH; CO_2 is given off.
4. Alpha-ketoglutarate is decaroboxylized and dehydrogenated; CO_2 is given off.
5. Phosphorylation occurs and guanosine triphosphate (GTP) is produced.
6. Oxidation occurs in which FAD is the hydrogen receptor.
7. Malate is formed.
8. Malate is converted to oxaloacetate, concluding the cycle.

Note: 30-32 adenosine tri-phosphates (ATPs) are produced from the oxidation of one molecule of glucose.

Excretion

The removal of waste products from the body is excretion. For solid products, the final destination is the terminal end of the rectum, known as the anus; contents are propelled via muscular reflex. Feces exit the anus and are composed of undigested material including fiber, bile pigments, and other undigested waste products. Urea is filtered by the kidneys and removed from the body in the form of liquid urine.

Renal

Renal System

The kidneys are the primary component of the renal system. The kidneys are a pair of bean-shaped organs responsible for maintaining fluid and electrolyte balance within the body and also contribute to the production of red blood cells. The kidneys filter using nephrons and rid the body of waste products or urea. The kidneys are also involved in blood pressure regulation through the release of renin. Renin is involved in the renin angiotensin aldosterone system, which controls blood volume. Other components of the urinary system include the bladder, ureters, and urethra. The ureters transport the urine to the bladder. The bladder is the pouch that holds the urine. The urethra is the structure that carries urine out of the body for excretion.

Metabolic Acidosis and Alkalosis

These conditions are related to kidney function. The kidneys function as a filter in part to maintain acid-base balance within the body. Metabolic acidosis results when there is too much acid in the bloodstream, thus lowering the pH. In this scenario the kidneys have increased production of hydrogen or failed to remove hydrogen, and the result is an increase in carbonic acid. Increased blood acidity will prompt the lungs to increase respiration rate. Metabolic alkalosis results when the pH is too high because of inadequate hydrogen present or the retention of too much bicarbonate (base). The result is slowed breathing in an effort to retain more carbon dioxide.

Pulmonary

Pulmonary System

The pulmonary system is responsible for gas exchange; we breathe oxygen and exhale carbon dioxide. We breathe air in through the nose, and air travels via the trachea into the lungs. The lungs are complex and composed of bronchi, bronchioles, and alveoli, and cilia. The main site of gas exchange is in the alveoli sacs, and cilia are "hairlike" extrusions that play a role in the removal of foreign bodies by facilitating the movement of mucus into the gastrointestinal tract. Breathing in air is a result of the contraction of the diaphragm. The pulmonary arteries transport blood rich in carbon dioxide to the lungs, where it is expelled, and oxygen is absorbed. Oxygenated blood can then be pumped throughout the body. The lungs also play a metabolic role such as helping to maintain pH balance, and the lungs are the site of conversion of angiotensin I to angiotensin II (involved in blood pressure regulation).

Respiratory Acidosis and Alkalosis

If breathing is impaired, gas exchange can be affected. Decreased ventilation or slowed breathing can cause a buildup of carbon dioxide. Too much carbon dioxide may result in the blood becoming too acidic, and this is called respiratory acidosis. When this occurs, the kidneys work to rid the body of excess acid. Respiratory alkalosis can also occur as blood pH rises due to excessive carbonic acid loss. Alkalosis may occur from hyperventilation; the kidneys work to remove base from the body to bring pH into balance.

Cardiovascular

The heart plays the central role in the functioning of the cardiovascular system, but the cardiovascular system is composed of a vast network of blood vessels that run like a series of roads and highways throughout the body. Arteries transport blood away from the heart, and veins return blood to the heart (e.g., the pulmonary vein brings oxygenated blood to the heart from the lungs). Oxygenated blood and nutrients can be pumped to other parts of the body, while the blood containing carbon dioxide travels to the lungs for removal. The heart is actually a muscle, and contraction results from electrical impulses. The heart's anatomy consists of different chambers: the right ventricle, left ventricle, left atrium, and right atrium. The right atrium and right ventricle are separated by the tricuspid valve. The left atrium and left ventricle are separated by the mitral valve. The pulmonary valve is the gatekeeper for blood that will flow to the lungs, and the aortic valve is the gatekeeper for the aorta.

Neurological

The brain and spinal cord are the primary components of the body's central nervous system. The brain has three main parts: the cerebrum, the cerebellum, and the brainstem, but it can be further subdivided into lobes. The brainstem connects the brain to the spinal cord. The spinal cord acts as the highway between the body and the brain—it transports signals to and from the brain. The brain lobes include the frontal lobe, which controls areas such as speech and behavior. The occipital lobe controls sight, the parietal lobe is involved in speech, and the temporal lobe is involved in memory and hearing. Located within the brain are also the hypothalamus and the pituitary gland. The hypothalamus controls hunger and thirst, and it also controls the pituitary gland. The pituitary gland is the regulator of our endocrine system and secretes many important hormones. Specifically, thyroid-stimulating hormone and human growth hormone come from the pituitary gland.

Musculoskeletal

In part, we can attribute our ability to move, walk, and run to our musculoskeletal system. Although the brain signals the body, bones, muscles, and ligaments provide the physical means to carry about the movement. The adult body contains 206 bones, whereas infants and children actually have more bones. As growth occurs, the bones fuse together. If some of our bones were already fused, growth would be limited. Bones do more than just provide structure and protection, although these are primary functions of the skeletal system. Bones also store calcium, which is necessary for many other bodily functions, and they house bone marrow, where red blood cell production takes place. Bones are connected to each other at hinges called joints. Ligaments help anchor the bones together, and tendons connect muscle to bone. Cartilage is also present to serve as a lubricator between bone surfaces. Skeletal muscles, which are attached to the tendons, are ultimately responsible for initiating movement.

Reproductive

The reproductive system is responsible for reproducing, and the contributing structures differ in males and females. In females, the vagina, cervix, uterus, fallopian tubes, and ovaries are primary. In males, the penis, testes, and prostate gland are involved in the reproductive process. The testes make sperm and produce the hormone testosterone. The prostate provides fluid to aid the sperm during their journey. The penis is responsible for delivering the sperm to the female for fertilization of the egg. The sperm and ejaculate enter the female through the vagina. Eggs and hormones are produced and released by the ovaries; fertilization occurs in the fallopian tubes. Once fertilized, the egg travels to the uterus, where it implants and remains until birth. Unlike males, who can continuously produce sperm, females are born with a set number of eggs and do not produce any beyond the fetal stage. The number and viability of eggs decrease as the female ages.

Nutrition Requirements and Health Promotion and Disease Prevention

The World Health Organization defines epidemiology as "the study of the distribution and determinants of health-related states or events (including disease) and the application of this study to the control of diseases and other health problems." Thus, epidemiology really looks at what conditions affect our health and impact disease. Organizations and individuals that study epidemiology, seek to determine factors that may contribute to our health. To impact and reduce disease (and thus improve our health), it is essential to know what leads to health problems. Although epidemiology is important in many aspects of health care, it is also important for nutrition-related problems. We know many factors such as income and cultural norms can affect our nutrition status, whereas factors such as gender and race influence our risk factors for certain diseases. Being aware of these determinants can help dietitians make better choices in providing nutrition intervention for our patients and the community.

Education, Communication and Technology

Targeted Setting/Clientele

In-Service Education

Facilities and organizations should strive to provide an environment of ongoing education for employees, volunteers, and student interns. In-services and frequent education are part of a more comprehensive training programming. Training does not end after the two-day orientation period; effective training is continuous. In-services are beneficial for employees and other workers to reinforce priorities, review goals, and set new objectives. These meetings also provide an avenue to share new information, educate, and serve to remind employees of proper workplace behavior. Whereas some in-services may focus on quality assurance and risk reduction, others may provide diversity training.

Patient/Client Counseling

The objective of the counseling session is to impart information and education to the patient. In doing so, the patient or caregivers must also provide you with necessary information. The dietitian should seek to establish a working relationship with the client. Building trust is important, and judgment should be avoided, but professional honesty is necessary. The client should feel comfortable sharing information about his or her life that affects nutrition status. If in a hospital setting, family and friends may be present, and the patient may feel uncomfortable about counseling during this time. The dietitian should ask the patient who may be present during the interview and seek to establish a comfortable atmosphere for the patient to speak. Asking open-ended questions and careful listening while showing empathy will help the dietitian gain a better understanding of the challenges affecting the client. During the communication process, the dietitian should be mindful and respectful of cultural differences. The nutrition education message should be delivered in a respectful manner that seeks to involve the client in the decision-making process.

Group Education

Group education occurs when more than one person is present for education or counseling. This may occur in the form of a class or a smaller gathering. Group educating provides an opportunity for many people facing the same challenges to be together and learn from one another. For example, diabetes education classes provide a setting where newly diagnosed diabetics can interact with others who are in the same situation. This setting not only provides the necessary education but also lends support. Of course, there are also downsides to group education classes. Some members of the group may not feel comfortable sharing information in front of the group. This should be respected. Some individuals may also benefit from individual education in addition to the group setting. Also, the group setting limits individual education, so specific needs are best handled in a one-on-one setting.

Goals and Objectives

Goal setting is part of the Nutrition Care Process (NCP). Goal setting is not only for the dietitian to measure whether objectives are met, but setting goals is also important for the client. Ideally, the dietitian will set goals with the client (or the caregiver if the client is unable to participate in the process). Why is this important? When goals are set, the client has something measurable toward which to work. Along with setting goals, the dietitian and client should discuss how to reach those goals. With this framework, the stakeholders in the process know where they are going and how they will get there. Goals should be measurable, and a time period for achieving should be specified.

Goals are not objectives set in stone; they can be changed or altered to better meet the needs of the client and to coincide with clinical objectives.

Goals may also apply to other situations; the dietitian may set goals in his or her workplace with the employer, or the dietitian may be the employer and set goals with his or her organization. When setting goals, it is important to involve the stakeholders—those who have a stake in the organization. It is important to consider factors and objectives that are important to partners and others who are involved. Otherwise, setting objectives may prove fruitless.

Needs Assessment

Before the dietitian begins educating, he or she must understand the needs of the individual or needs of the group. An understanding of needs will help the dietitian develop a framework for the education plan. Without first conducting a needs assessment, the dietitian will not have a baseline from which to work. It is important to assess the current knowledge base of the client or clients to direct the education appropriately. A newly diagnosed diabetic may have a limited understanding of diabetes, whereas a long-standing diabetic may have more knowledge. At the same time, the long-standing diabetic may have a limited understanding of how diet affects his or her diabetes, so it is important to avoid making assumptions. A thorough needs assessment will evaluate knowledge and the ability to comply, along with other pertinent details that may affect the education plan and outcomes.

Content

Before conducting an education session, the dietitian must first plan the content of the class or counseling session. What will happen in the class? How will it be conducted? What type of education materials will you provide to the participants? These are all questions that must be answered during the preparation stage. First, consider who will teach the class? Will you teach the class, or will you invite a guest speaker from the community? For instance, suppose you are conducting a class on cardiovascular health. Perhaps you could invite an exercise physiologist to discuss incorporating exercise into a healthy lifestyle. What type of visual aids will be used? Although hearing a speaker provides information, incorporating the visual senses is often helpful in a classroom environment. Options include using PowerPoint, a whiteboard, and food models to reinforce the message. If you are using a program such as PowerPoint, the content should be easy to read (font at least 24) and not too cluttered (leave white space). Will you provide handouts for take-home reference? Handouts can be a useful tool, but they should be easy to read and concise. Adequate planning and use of resources are necessary in facilitating an education session.

Evaluation Criteria

The purpose of the class is to educate, so clearly you want to know if the goals of the session have been met. Having your participants evaluate the speaker, materials, presentation, and overall class effectiveness is one such way to determine success. There is always room for improvement, and unless the educational session is evaluated, you cannot assess *where* to improve or *how* to improve. You could ask the audience if they felt the presentation was useful, but many people would feel uncomfortable publicly commenting. Providing a questionnaire to the class will offer you valuable feedback. With the feedback provided, you can improve upon elements that were effective for the participants and delete or change aspects that were not helpful. You can also determine the types of programs or topics the audience would like to see in the future. To encourage participation, the form should be relatively short and easy to read.

Budget Development

First, you must consider whether you have the funds for your program offering and whether you wish to use those funds on the program under consideration. Most likely, your department or project will have a specific amount of funds allocated. You must decide how to use those funds to meet your objectives, and this information should be detailed in the form of a budget for your educational program. Why budget? A budget is really a plan for how money will be spent. Without a proper plan, you could use all of your funds in one area and not have enough money for another area. Planning and allocating funds appropriately while involving stakeholders in the budgetary process will help avoid a negative financial outcome.

Program Promotion

If you are putting time, money, and effort into creating an educational program, you want people to attend, so they must know the program is taking place and be informed of details such as date and time, location, and the purpose of the session. Who are you trying to reach (target audience), and how will you reach these individuals? If you are offering a diabetes education class, you can consider contacting local physician groups and providing them with the details. In turn, they may refer their patients. You can also have flyers distributed or displayed in doctor's offices, hospitals, and senior centers advertising the program. Perhaps you already have a list of potential attendees from your patient list. You can reach out via mail or email to these individuals with program details. Another avenue to advertise is through participation in health fairs. This provides an opportunity to share with the public any programs or other offerings your organization may sponsor.

Educational Readiness

Considering Educational Readiness

Why is educational readiness important? Being ready to change or open to change certainly improves the odds of behavior change and helps improve the chances your message will be received. If your client or patient is not ready to make some life-altering changes, it likely will not happen. Although you the dietitian may have a wonderful plan to help the client meet your goals, you must consider the goals of the client and his or her openness to being educated and modifying behavior. Assessing education readiness in your client is an important first step. If he or she is not ready, you may take steps that will promote readiness. The Health Belief Model suggests a person's attitudes toward an illness or disease coupled with the perceived effectiveness of the treatment will ultimately predict whether change will occur. Does the patient take his or her disease seriously? Do the negative outcomes of the disease concern them? Does the patient have confidence that what you are proposing (nutrition intervention) will improve his or her outcomes? This is one model, and certainly behavioral change is rarely this simple. People are often resistant to change; many contributing factors should be considered when behavior change is needed.

Grief Model

This model was originally designed to explore the stages of grief prior to death, but it also has implications for behavior change. For instance, a newly diagnosed cardiovascular disease patient who has recently had a heart attack might go through the stages described in the grief model. The stages are as follows:

- Denial—the patient tells him- or herself that heart disease is no big deal. It is hard to accept the reality of having had a heart attack and the implications that come with having heart disease.
- Anger—the patient gets mad about the situation. He or she focuses on the unfairness of the situation. He or she might consider a person they know who eats whatever they want and never exercises but did not have a heart attack!
- Bargaining—this is when the patient might say, "I will exercise a couple of times per week and try to eat a little better." There really is not commitment to change at this point.
- Depression—the patient realizes he or she will have to do more than make small changes. This disease is life changing; depression may result from this change-of-life event.
- Acceptance—at this stage the patient either resolves to make real changes or accepts the reality of what may result from not making health changes.

Human Behavior and Change Management Theory

There are many models that address behavior change, and two are described here.

Lewin's Change Management Model can be applied to changes in organizations, but it can also be applied to individuals. This model takes a three-step approach to change. The first step is to unfreeze. In this initial step, you the dietitian should open the door to change by explaining why change is necessary and the benefits associated with change. The second step is change. At this point, behavioral changes begin to occur over a period of time. The last step is refreezing. At this stage, changes have been implemented and have become commonplace. You want to this behavioral trend to continue and become commonplace.

The Theory of Planned Behavior proposed by Ajzen and Fishbein proposes that our beliefs and attitudes, coupled with the beliefs of influencing people, will predict behavior. From a health perspective, the patient would consider his or her disease and take into account how close family members might feel about treatment or intervention.

Theories abound that try to predict behavior and explain behavioral change. In reality, behavior change is a complicated process that involves emotions, desires, finances, physical and mental limitations, as well as social aspects. There are many influences that impact our behavior, and the dietitian must carefully consider these areas when approaching change.

Communication

Communication is more than just one person talking. Communication is an exchange of ideas and information among people. The manner in which we communicate can affect the outcome of situations, work projects, or interventions. Perhaps one of the most important aspects of communication is actually listening. You need to hear and process what others are saying to be an effective communicator. Ask questions during the exchange and repeat responses in the form of paraphrasing showing there is an acknowledgement of understanding. The nonverbal cues that you send also impact the communication process. Appearing with arms crossed and a scowl on the face sends a negative message; alternatively, eye contact and nodding are encouraging and show understanding. Also, consider your tone of voice. You may say something kind or encouraging, but if the tone is rough or sarcastic, the message will not be received as perhaps you had intended. It is also important to provide feedback in a nonjudgmental manner.

Group Process

Effective Group Characteristics

Groups of people work together to achieve a specific objective. How that group operates together can impact the success of outcomes. Groups that work together should have clear goals. Members should be committed to the task at hand and willing to participate. Effective teams should communicate often, openly, and honestly. Team members should promote unity, and a sense of trust is important. Members should know and understand their roles and feel comfortable carrying out their responsibilities. People working in groups often produces interesting, unpredictable outcomes. The Risky Shift Phenomenon says group decision-making tends to result in decisions that are riskier or more extreme than they might make if acting alone. The opposite of greater risk-taking behavior also results in that groups are afraid their actions will adversely impact the group, so they take fewer risks. This phenomenon could have both positive and negative outcomes depending on the situation.

Groupthink

Groupthink is a common phenomenon that occurs when people go along with the group. Perhaps no one wants "to rock the boat" or dissent. Groupthink can have negative consequences in that poor decisions may result. Most groups have a combination of outgoing and dominating personalities combined with more reserved individuals. It is important that everyone has a chance to be heard, and there are steps that should be taken to ensure the team is performing at an optimal level.

Groupthink can be limited with the following actions:

- Assign a devil's advocate to challenge decisions.
- Encourage open dialogue, questions, and concerns.
- Seek outside opinions.
- As a leader, do not be overbearing.
- Explore and establish alternatives plans—do not decide on one method or plan at the onset.

Teach Classes

Culinary demonstrations could be used when the audience has limited knowledge of cooking or when the audience has a specific interest in cooking. The demonstration would be tailored to the skill level of the audience. If you have a group needing to prepare quick, yet healthy family meals, your demo would illustrate that approach. Rather if you have an audience that is less restrained by time and more focused on other culinary aspects, you might focus on meals that require more time and skill. Perhaps a group member has a favorite recipe that he or she would like to "make healthy." This would be a good cooking illustration.

Grocery store tours can be incorporated into a class and are an effective means to discuss specific foods and read food labels. Often, one can get overwhelmed at the endless choices in the grocery store aisles. The grocery tour enables the dietitian to promote specific, healthier choices while also communicating items that should be limited or avoided. Class members can begin the tour with a "grocery list" and use this as the basis for teaching.

Interviewing

Interviewing is how you gather information, and your approach will impact the type and usefulness of the feedback. To provide targeted intervention, you want to gather quality information that helps you assess the patient. Open-ended questions or statements are more likely to provide you with the most information as compared to closed-ended questions. The following is an example of an open-ended statement that asks for information: "Tell me about some challenges you have faced in trying to lose weight." This type of approach will provide you with more detailed information than a closed-ended question, such as, "Have you had challenges losing weight?" This type of question is not particularly helpful because most likely the patient is seeking the dietitian's expertise due to challenges. As the dietitian, you need to know what challenges are being faced so you can provide the best education and intervention strategies. Use caution when using leading questions. As the name suggests, such questions can lead the client to a specific answer that may not be the most accurate.

Counseling

Motivational Counseling

Motivational counseling may also be referred to as motivational interviewing. Motivational counseling is an approach one takes to counseling. A key part of behavior change is the motivation to do so, and as a nutrition counselor, part of your job is to help motivate. Rather than talking at someone, which may result in one-way communication, motivational interviewing involves a healthy, productive exchange of information. As part of motivational interviewing you not only provide feedback in the form of education, but you listen to what is being communicated by the client. In turn, you show empathy and understanding for the challenges and triumphs the client is facing. In many ways, motivational interviewing can be thought of as a pointed conversation that facilitates behavior change.

Cognitive Behavioral Therapy

Cognitive Behavioral Therapy (CBT) can be used in many different types of counseling situations. Dietitians can successfully employ this approach as well in addressing nutrition-related issues such as obesity and some eating disorders. CBT can be used to help patients "unlearn" certain unhealthy behaviors. For instance, if you are addressing someone who eats when he or she feels stressed or unhappy, it is important that this person learn to disassociate feelings and food. The way we feel, in reality, does not necessitate the need to eat. More likely, eating when we are stressed or upset has become a habit. With CBT, you train yourself not to associate food with feelings. Rather food should be associated with true hunger and sustaining life; the emotions should be dealt with in more constructive ways.

Methods of Communication

Verbal and Nonverbal

Verbal communication is what we speak and how we say things. When speaking, we want to speak clearly and thoughtfully using a nonjudgmental and non-condescending tone of voice. Just as important as our verbal communication is our nonverbal communication. We do not always communicate with our words; sometimes our body language sends messages as well. When we cross our arms, we portray a closed-off mentality rather than someone who encourages communication. Our facial expressions also send positive or negative messages to our clients and coworkers. It is also important to make eye contact rather than looking around when speaking and listening to someone. Eye contact signals that you are paying attention and hearing what is being communicated. As trusted health-care professionals who spend time interacting with patients, it is important that we communicate appropriately to be the most effective at our jobs.

Written

Just as one should use care with spoken word, the same is true for written communications. When writing, there is a record of what you have communicated, and your words and approach should be thoughtful and professional.

Although emails have become casual over time, remember you are a professional. Emails can offer an avenue for quick exchanges but take care to maintain a professional tone and image when writing. One should seek to avoid spelling and grammatical errors. As always, patient privacy should be maintained with any form of communication.

As a dietitian, you may be asked to prepare reports for work or write grant proposals to obtain funding. Writing skills are important in these endeavors, and your writing is reflective of you as a dietitian. As with all forms of written communication, a thorough, professional approach is expected.

Media

Dietitians have more outlets for communication than ever before. To communicate our nutrition message, we can use a variety of media including websites, magazines, flyers, billboards, and social media. Print media is still used today even with the influence of the Internet. Not all individuals rely on the Internet for the exchange of all information, so print media still has a place. To advertise a nutrition class, you may want to use flyers and hang them in strategic locations. You may use pamphlets and business cards to provide information about your business. To reach a greater audience, you may establish a web page that can be continuously updated where people can go to find detailed information about your practice or class offerings. Social media is yet another tool that allows dietitians to reach an audience. Many use social media to quickly provide updates, education, and announcements.

Measurement of Learning

Formative and Summative Evaluations

Both summative and formative measures are used to evaluate learning. Formative evaluations provide continuous feedback about how a class or counseling is proceeding. Having real-time data to assess can help the practitioner make changes in the plan or approach. Alternatively, summative evaluations measure learning at the end of an educational period. For example, if you were conducting a series of classes and you evaluated outcomes at the end of that series, this is a type of summative evaluation. If you measured at the end of each individual class, you would be using formative evaluation.

Evaluation of Effectiveness of Educational Plan

The logic model is one method to evaluate the effectiveness of your educational plan. Logic models can demonstrate and illustrate a framework for how your educational plan will operate. Logic models use pictures to show a sequence of events in a plan. Logic models may have different steps illustrated, but the following provides some useful components. First, you should explain the purpose of the program or why you are conducting the class. For instance, why are you offering a diabetes education class? What are you hoping to accomplish with this educational program? Next, you may illustrate the resources and challenges anticipated. A resource might be subject-matter experts, whereas a challenge might be regular class attendance for participants. Then, you should illustrate what you will do in the class or educational series. Finally, you should illustrate outcomes and detail whether you were successful in meeting your program goals. If your goals are not met, what areas of the logic model would you change or adjust to improve the effectiveness of your program? Regardless of which model or approach you use, evaluating your educational plan provides valuable feedback for improvement.

Documentation and HIPAA

The medical record is a legal document, and it should be treated as such. Information contained in the medical record is confidential. HIPAA is the Health Insurance Portability and Accountability Act and was enacted in 1996. As electronic systems were becoming the norm, HIPAA was enacted to protect the public by putting security and privacy rules into place. HIPAA also gives patients the right to view their medical records.

Beyond the legalities, the medical record houses pertinent health information about the patient. Healthcare professionals document or record their interactions and interventions with the patient; documentation provides a record of care that helps ensure continuity. The medical record also serves as tool to communicate with other professionals. With proper documentation, the plan of care for an individual should be evident and clear to others reading the documentation. As a dietitian, you will also document your plan of care. Dietitians should adopt the Nutrition Care Process and use standardized language when documenting.

Orientation and Training Program

Orientation programs may be conducted at the onset of a program or employment. Orientation programs take many forms, but they serve to orient the participant or employee to the program or workplace. Training programs differ in that they seek to provide ongoing education or training. Training programs can be effective in the workplace when teaching new skills. Ongoing training can be essential in the workplace to reinforce information and to enhance job skills.

Electronic Health Records

Benefits and Concerns Associated with Electronic Health Records

Merriam-Webster defines informatics as, "the collection, classification, storage, retrieval, and dissemination of recorded knowledge." The electronic health record is an example of informatics in use. There are advantages to the electronic medical record (EMR) compared to a paper record. Whereas only one paper record may exist, the EMR allows for access by multiple individuals in multiple locations. This may help improve access to information and continuity of care. Of course, with this ease of access also comes privacy concerns. Confidentiality of health information remains paramount; organizations and providers are required to take steps that protect health information.

Telehealth and Remote Health Monitoring

More and more, alternatives to traditional health-care settings are being introduced and are known as telehealth. Telehealth options offer patients and providers the ability to interact remotely without being in the same physical location. Telehealth provides convenience and can also promote access to providers in underserved or rural areas. Telehealth sessions are often conducted by video but could also be conducted by phone. Remote health monitoring programs collect health information (while the patient is at home or work), and the data is transmitted electronically to another location (the provider). Like telehealth, remote health monitoring systems provide greater access for those who are unable to visit a provider. Telehealth may help eliminate the need for individuals to take time off work or travel great distances. Barriers such as limited provider access or lack of transportation can be somewhat alleviated with remote health monitoring. Telehealth services and remote health monitoring offer the opportunity for improving health in some populations that might otherwise be underserved.

Food Service Management Software

Dietitians may use nutrient analysis software and databases to help analyze diets for adequacy. The United States Department of Agriculture (USDA) provides a free nutrient database, and several commercial databases are available for purchase.

Food service operations often employ software to facilitate business activities. Software may be used to track inventory and for costing and ordering, menu development, and scheduling. Healthcare facilities may also use the preceding types of software but in addition often require software that helps manage therapeutic diets.

PUBLIC POLICY DISCUSSION AND FAMILIARITY WITH THE LEGISLATIVE PROCESS

As health-care professionals, dietitians may wish to advocate for their patients and their profession. Citizens can offer a voice by contacting your elected representatives in matters involving funding and legislation that can impact dietician practice or health care in general.

The steps in the legislative process are as follows:

1. A bill is proposed or introduced.
2. The bill goes to committee; it may die in committee or may move forward.
3. A hearing or vote may be scheduled.
4. If the bill passes, it can be moved to the other chamber (Senate or House depending on its origin).
5. A similar process is followed in this chamber (the bill goes to committee).
6. If there are changes to the original bill, the changes must be resolved and agreed upon by both chambers.
7. The final bill will be voted on by the House and Senate.
8. The president has the option to sign the bill into law or veto.

Research Applications

Research

Descriptive: Descriptive research is intended to describe a problem or event rather than making cause-and-effect predictions. The case study method is an example of descriptive research.

Analytical: Analytical research attempts to establish a cause-and-effect relationship. Regression analysis is one such example of an analytical research method.

Qualitative: Qualitative research generally involves thoughts and opinions rather than facts; it is often conducted as initial research that then leads to further research.

Quantitative: Quantitative research involves facts and figures (numbers).

Research Process

Research will generally be conducted by following the scientific method. The following are some basic steps involved in research:

1. Define the problem or area to be studied.
2. Gather information (one method is through literature review).
3. Establish hypothesis (the hypothesis is what you are trying to prove or disprove).
4. Design and conduct an experiment (test the hypothesis and collect experimental data; the study should be repeated for accuracy).
5. Analyze and interpret data (may use statistical analysis).
6. Discus results (how do the results compare with other studies; was the hypothesis proved or disproved).

The Institutional Research Board (IRB) is a governing body that exists to protect the welfare of human research subjects by instituting ethical standards; furthermore, the IRB ensures applicable laws are followed.

Application of Statistical Analysis

Experimental and Observational Statistical Study

An experimental study isolates a variable to be studied and then further identifies other variables that may impact the variable of study. From a nutrition perspective, let's suppose we wanted to study how the intake of certain foods affect cholesterol levels. Cholesterol would be our primary study variable, and other variables included in the study might be fiber and beef. The object of the study is to determine how the other variables affect cholesterol levels. An observational study does not control the variables in the same manner. A survey is an example of an observational study.

Descriptive and Inferential Statistics

Descriptive statistics are summaries of data and may be presented in graphical or table form. Some terminology associated with descriptive statistics include the mean, median, and mode. The mean is the average of a set of numbers, the median is the number in the middle of a numerical, ordered set, and the mode is the number that appears most often the data set. The standard deviation indicates how spread out the numbers are from the average and is also the square root of the variance.

Inferential statistics infers information from a data sample. For instance, if you want information on dietary intake for a particular state or metropolitan area, it would be unrealistic to question every individual. Rather, a sample of the population would be interviewed or studied, and conclusions could be drawn from that sample.

Regression Analysis

Regression analysis looks at the relationship between two variables (simple regression). The dependent variable is generally denoted by the letter Y, and Y is the variable we will predict (the outcome of Y depends on X). X is the independent variable and will be used to predict Y. Regression analysis will yield an output that can be interpreted. The R value tells us if there is a linear relationship. R^2 tells us whether our regression line mimics reality. The higher the value, the better. The p-value gives us an indication as to whether the results occurred by chance. A lower p-value supports a valid result. For example, a p-value of 0.019 indicates there is only a 1.9% chance the result is a fluke. A cut-off p-value of less than 0.05 is often used in research to indicate significance. The standard error is another output and measures whether our sample is representative of the overall population. If our sample does not reflect reality, this makes it difficult to draw accurate conclusions.

Analysis, Interpretation, and Integration of Evidence-Based Research Findings

As dietitians, it is imperative to put evidence-based research into practice because our message should be based on sound, peer-reviewed research, and scientific principles. The Academy of Nutrition and Dietetics describe evidence-based practice as follows: "Evidence-based dietetics practice is the use of systematically reviewed scientific evidence in making food and nutrition practice decisions by integrating best available evidence with professional expertise and client values to improve outcomes." The incorporation of evidence-based practice guidelines into our everyday practice can help improve patient care, lends credibility, and can lead to better outcomes. Part of the Nutrition Care Process is to support and utilize evidence-based research and guidelines in the practice of dietetics. The Academy of Nutrition and Dietetics provides resources to incorporate sound principles into practice; an example is the Evidence Analysis Library (EAL). The EAL provides reliable, peer-reviewed information for dietitians to access and apply to practice.

Presentation of Research Data and Reporting Research Findings

Data should be presented in a way that is easy to read and understand. In research, you may be reporting a tremendous amount of data. Text may be used to convey some information, especially qualitative information. Quantitative information is often best displayed in a table or chart.

Research published in a peer-reviewed journal will generally follow a typical format that includes the following components:

1. Abstract: overviews the research
2. Introduction: tells you why the research is being done
3. Literature review: reviews existing literature on the subject
4. Methods: describes how the research was conducted
5. Results: includes findings of the research
6. Discussion: includes interpretation and implications of research
7. Conclusions: describes final comments about results and need for further research
8. References

Nutrition Care for Individuals and Groups

Screening and Assessment

Purpose

The purpose of nutrition screening is to determine if an individual has a nutritional risk. Screening should be initiated before beginning the nutrition care process. In a hospital setting, the screening should take place as soon as possible; the requirement is typically within 24 hours of admission. Because it is not financially feasible or efficient to assess every single patient in the healthcare setting, a screening tool helps to determine those who may benefit from an in-depth assessment from the dietitian. Screening tools will vary depending on the setting or facility, and in the hospital, the initial screening may be conducted by nursing staff. Each facility will determine the screening criteria, but certain diagnoses or indicators may trigger a nutrition referral. Potential triggers from a nutrition referral may include malnutrition, overweight or obesity, underweight, laboratory data, food insecurity, recent/unexplained weight loss, diabetes, or heart disease.

Parameters and Limitations

Nutrition screening cannot determine risk; it only prompts an assessment by the dietitian and suggests the potential for a problem. The goal of screening is to identify those who would benefit from nutrition intervention, but not every individual who is screened will be properly identified. Likewise, individuals who are identified via a screening tool may not be at nutritional risk. Suppose the dietitian receives a referral for a child who is slightly underweight. Upon further assessment, the dietitian determines that intake is adequate, and growth is consistent. Both parents are lean, and it is likely the child has a genetic tendency to be lean. Although the child is not at nutritional risk, this could not be determined with a degree of certainly unless an assessment was conducted. Furthermore, nutritional needs can change. Perhaps while a patient is hospitalized, he/she has a mild stroke and subsequently experiences swallowing problems. Although it is possible that the initial indicators did not warrant a nutritional referral, the situation has changed, and this patient would benefit from nutrition intervention. In addition, screenings often rely on verbal feedback from the patient or family members. Language barriers resulting from cultural differences may inhibit the ability of the screener to obtain the correct information. Having qualified translators available can help alleviate this limitation.

Methodology

There is not a standardized screening process or tool that facilities or providers are required to use. Each office, community health center, or hospital can develop their own screening tool, and the tool/form can be individualized depending on the setting. A screening tool for the hospital may be different from a community health center screening tool. The purpose of screening is to identify individuals who have a potential nutrition-related problem such as malnutrition. Screenings will frequently look at the history of recent, unintended weight loss as well as the significance of weight loss; both instances may point to malnutrition. In general, screening tools should be uncomplicated and easy to use by most disciplines, and they should be reliable.

Participation in Interdisciplinary Nutrition Screening Teams

Facilities and community health centers will have a formal nutrition screening process in place. Often, dietitians are not the providers responsible for the screening process. In hospitals, this duty often falls to the nursing staff to address upon the patient being admitted to the hospital. During the hospital stay, physicians or speech/language pathologists may refer to the dietitian after a triggering event. For instance, a physician may initiate a referral based on a postoperative patient needing parenteral nutrition. Likewise, a speech pathologist may determine that a patient has swallowing difficulty and request a nutrition consult. In the community health setting, referrals may be initiated by nursing staff, non-registered dietitian Women, Infants, and Children (WIC) Program staff, and social workers. The social worker may note food insecurity in a home, or he/she may note that a child appears thin/undernourished. The WIC staff may encounter a child who is severely overweight or an infant with failure to thrive. Such concerns will likely initiate a referral to the dietitian for further assessment.

Prioritizing Nutrition Risk

Prioritizing nutrition risk is important to focus the resources where most needed. Resources may include dollars and staffing, both of which are limited. Directing resources towards the greatest needs is an efficient way of operating. When conducting a nutrition screening, individuals and groups at the highest risk should receive the highest priority, and individuals at a lower risk will be categorized appropriately. Individuals who are at low risk may not be assessed immediately and may require no intervention, whereas someone at moderate risk may warrant closer observation. A patient at high risk, perhaps an individual with extreme, unintentional weight loss, would require intervention and daily, ongoing monitoring. Each facility or program will have its own methods/criteria to prioritize nutrition risk. Screening tools will differ among entities; long-term care facilities, acute care facilities, and community agencies should use the tools most appropriate for the setting. Essentially, prioritizing the nutrition risk helps to ensure that those who most need intervention get the appropriate focus.

Dietary Intake Assessment, Analysis, and Documentation

Nutrition Care Process

The first step in the Nutrition Care Process (NCP) is the nutrition assessment. The assessment phase is the investigation; the dietitian obtains information needed to make a nutrition diagnosis (or determines that there is no diagnosis). Information gathered during the assessment can include height, weight, food intake, laboratory test results, medications/herbal remedies, physical observations, family medical history, and personal medical history. The dietitian may gather information from the patient, family members, and the medical record. Observations and thoughtful questioning can be useful in gathering the necessary feedback. During the assessment, it is important to compare the nutrition indicators against the appropriate comparative standard. The Dietary Reference Intakes (DRIs) are an example of a comparative standard that might be used. According to the Academy of Nutrition and Dietetics, when choosing a comparative reference standard, it is important to consider the practice setting, population characteristics, and disease state or severity. If you choose the wrong standard to reference, your nutrition diagnosis, prescription, and outcomes could be adversely affected.

Dietary Intake Assessment and Analysis

Assessing dietary intake gives the dietitian a snapshot into the client's eating practices; this will be useful for assessment and counseling. A variety of methods to obtain intake may be used including a 24-hour recall, a food frequency questionnaire, or a food diary. A 24-hour recall is when the client relays the foods/beverages eaten during a 24-hour period. The recall period should be a typical day's intake. For example, a family gathering for a holiday meal may not be reflective of typical dietary intake. Recalls have limitations in that clients may not remember everything eaten and drank, or they may be unable to accurately describe the portions consumed. The food frequency questionnaire asks about how often certain foods are eaten. For example, it may ask, "How many times per week do you eat green vegetables or fresh fruits?" The food diary is often more comprehensive than a recall or frequency questionnaire. The client keeps a journal of foods and drink consumed along with the amounts. This method tends to provide more accurate information if the client records in an accurate and timely manner. Once the food intake data are obtained, they may be compared to a standardized reference for analysis.

Medical and Family History

A patient's medical history and family history may put them at risk for nutrition problems either now or in the future. A person's medical diagnosis and nutritional status are often linked. For example, an individual diagnosed with type 2 diabetes would benefit from nutrition intervention, given the link between control of type 2 diabetes and dietary intake. In addition, having type 2 diabetes is a risk factor for heart disease. As another example, suppose you have a concerned client who is experiencing recent weight loss. When recording the client's medical history, you discover that the client had surgery a few weeks ago. The surgery may be a contributing factor to the weight loss and should prompt the need for further investigation. Without the medical history knowledge, a different, possibly incorrect conclusion may be reached. Family history may also put a client at risk for nutrition-related problems. A client with a family history of obesity and heart disease may benefit from a proactive, heart-healthy dietary approach. To gain the most relevant information, it is important to consider the overall health and well-being of a patient/client when assessing.

Obtain and Assess Physical Findings

Anthropometric Data

Using Anthropometric Data in Nutrition Assessment

Anthropometric data are cornerstones of the nutrition assessment. Anthropometry includes height, weight, and skinfold thickness. Head circumference measurements are used in children younger than 36 months of age. From the height and weight measurements, the dietitian will determine the ideal body weight, BMI, and percentage weight loss/gain. The ideal body weight (IBW) calculation has limitations and is best used in conjunction with clinical judgment, but as the name suggests, it indicates where a person's weight should ideally fall. Body mass index (BMI) compares height to weight and tells us if those numbers are in proportion. A particularly high or low BMI may signal the need for dietary intervention. Percentage weight loss calculations are used to determine the percentage of body weight that has been lost within a given period of time and may be indicative of a bigger problem.

Calculations for the Ideal Body Weight and Percentage Weight Loss

Ideal Body Weight:

Women: 100 pounds for 5 feet in height. Add 5 pounds for each inch over 5 feet.

For example, you have a patient who is a 5'4" tall and female. 100 lbs + 4 × 5 = 120 IBW.

Men: 106 pounds for 5 feet in height. Add 6 pounds for each inch over 5 feet.

For example, you have a patient who is 5'11" tall and male. 106 + 11 × 6 = 172 IBW.

Percentage Weight Loss:

Percentage weight loss = (usual weight – actual weight) / (usual weight) × 100

Suppose your patient typically weighs 135 lbs, but recent weight loss results in an actual weight of 125 lbs. The percentage weight loss is (135 – 125) / (135) × 100 = 7.4 % weight loss.

Body Mass Index (BMI)

The dietitian will calculate BMI to help determine if a patient's weight is appropriate for their height. Because of the risk factors associated with overweight and obesity, a greater emphasis is placed on achieving and maintaining a healthy weight. A BMI indicating overweight or obesity may signal a need for dietary intervention through a reduction in calories. BMI can also help a dietitian know if a patient is underweight and in need of additional nutritional supplements. For children and teens (ages 2–20), the BMI must be plotted on the appropriate percentile chart to determine if it is within the normal range.

BMI = weight (kg) / height $(m)^2$.

BMI = weight (lbs) / height $(in)^2 \times 703$.

Classifications for adults:

Underweight: less than 18.5.

Normal: 18.5–24.9.

Overweight: 25–29.

Obese: greater than 30.

Waist/Hip Ratio

The waist/hip ratio compares the circumference of the hips to the circumference of the waist. Care should be taken to ensure that the measurements are accurate. Proper measurement location is important; the waist should be measured at the narrowest area, and the hips should be measured at the widest area. The waist/hip w may help indicate if fat is localized in the abdominal area (apple-shaped individuals) or in the hips (pear-shaped individuals). Abdominal fat has been linked to an increased risk for cardiovascular disease, so this measurement can be an important anthropometric measurement. The World Health Organization indicates that a ratio greater than 9.0 in men and greater than 8.5 in women is indicative of obesity and may contribute to metabolic diseases.

Waist/hip ratio = waist circumference/hip circumference.

Nutrition-Focused Physical Exam

Physical observations can provide insight into one's nutritional status and should not be overlooked as part of the nutrition assessment. Physical signs can be indicative of malnutrition, overnutrition, and vitamin/mineral deficiencies. The level of alertness and patient's mood can provide insight into the ability or desire to eat. The dietitian should note the patient's overall appearance and whether they appear healthy, frail, or overweight. Observe for skin turgor/elasticity, which can be indicative of hydration status or edema. Dry skin hair health should be indicated because both characteristics can be related to vitamin deficiency or thyroid disease. Although thyroid disease is a medical diagnosis, it generally results in altered metabolism, which would be addressed by the dietitian. Oral health should be observed when possible; missing teeth, dentures, and mouth sores should be noted. Oral health information provides insight into the patient's ability to eat and chew without difficulty. Although physical findings are only one piece of the assessment puzzle, observations along with other data can help determine an appropriate nutrition diagnosis.

Intake and Output

Intake refers to foods and fluids going into the body, whereas output refers to what comes out in the form of urine and stools. Intake may be in the form of an oral diet, enteral nutrition, or parenteral nutrition. Intake may be recorded in the hospital if there is a concern that the patient is not consuming enough nutrients orally. In this case, calorie counts may be ordered, which are obtained by recording all food/drink intake from patient meals and snacks. Intake is also important for alternate nutrition such as enteral feedings. Although there will be a diet order indicating a prescribed amount of tube feeding, it is important to establish that the amount that is ordered is the amount that is actually received. Output may be important in assessing for dehydration and constipation.

Medication/Food Interactions

Medications have side effects, and sometimes those side effects have nutrition-related consequences. For example, chemotherapy medications may cause dry mouth and resulting mouth sores. This may have an adversely affect oral intake. Diuretics cause increased urination; hydration and electrolytes are important considerations with diuretic use. Various medications may have many other side effects including appetite loss, increased appetite, altered nutrient absorption, and gastrointestinal upset. In addition to potential nutrition-related complications, medications may also interact with foods causing decreased effectiveness or other problems. For example, Synthroid or levothyroxine taken for hypothyroidism should not be taken with calcium- or fiber-containing foods. Both can limit the absorption of the medication. The medication warfarin is a blood thinner sometimes used in the treatment of heart disease. Vitamin K can impact the effectiveness of warfarin; the intake of vitamin K does not have to be eliminated, but it should not be variable from day to day. The dietitian must understand how medications can affect the patient's nutritional status and how one's dietary intake can affect pharmacologic effectiveness. With this knowledge, an appropriate diet plan can be administered.

Obtain and Assess Biochemical Data, Diagnostic Tests, and Procedures

Hemoglobin and Hematocrit Laboratory Values

Measurements of hemoglobin (Hgb) and hematocrit (Hct) are often used to assess iron status. A low hemoglobin or hematocrit value can indicate iron deficiency anemia. Anemia may be caused by disease progression or poor nutrition; it is important to establish the cause. If the anemia is related to dietary intake, the dietitian can recommend iron-rich foods to help improve nutrition status. Meats such as fish, chicken, beef, and pork provide the best dietary option because the iron in meats is absorbed more readily than the iron in plant products. Not all patients consume meats; plants that offer good sources of iron include rice, dark-green vegetables, and beans. Combining iron-containing foods with a source of vitamin C such as juice or fruit will enhance absorption.

Normal ranges for Hgb and Hct:

Hemoglobin

Men: 14–18 g/dl

Women: 12–16 g/dl

Pregnancy: > 11 g/dl

HEMATOCRIT

Men: 42–52%

Women: 35–47%

Pregnancy: 33%

PREALBUMIN AND ALBUMIN

Both albumin and prealbumin are blood indicators that dietitians use to assess protein status. Albumin is produced in the liver; poor liver function and dehydration can affect the measure. The half-life of albumin is approximately 20 days. Assume a patient was admitted to the hospital and began a tube feeding. Albumin has been ordered, and the level is low despite adequate intake. Because of the long half-life of albumin, a low level is not indicative of the present state. Prealbumin is a better indicator and should be used. In addition, a body under stress may show low levels of albumin even if the patient is well fed. A normal albumin level is 3.5–5.0 g/dL. Prealbumin is also made in the liver and has a shorter half-life than albumin at approximately two days. Changes in status would be more apparent with the measurement of prealbumin versus measuring albumin. Like albumin, prealbumin is responsive to stress.

LABORATORY INDICATORS FOR KIDNEY FUNCTION

Blood urea nitrogen (BUN) and creatinine levels are indicative of kidney function. Both of these levels will be high in kidney disease and signify poor excretion by the kidneys. Abnormal laboratory test results may indicate acute kidney failure or chronic kidney failure. Other laboratory tests to monitor kidney function include sodium (Na), potassium (K), total calcium, and phosphorus.

Normal BUN levels: 5–20 mg/dL

Normal creatinine levels: 0.5–1.2 mg/dL

The estimated glomerular filtration rate (eGFR) provides an indication of how quickly the kidneys are able to filter waste products. The National Kidney Foundation classifies the stages of chronic kidney disease according to the eGFR. An eGFR of less than 15 mL/minute is indicative of kidney failure. At this point, dialysis or transplantation are the only treatment options.

IMPORTANCE OF CONSIDERING DIAGNOSTIC TESTS AND PROCEDURES

Laboratory data and other diagnostic tests and procedures can provide insight into one's medical status and nutrition status. A person's medical state can be affected by nutrition, and likewise the medical state can adversely affect one's nutrition status. The dietitian benefits from having a complete picture of the patient's health, and although these indicators are useful in the healthcare setting, clinical judgment must always be exercised. When assessing laboratory data, the dietitian must consider the many factors that may affect the test including nutrition status, hydration, and stress response. For example, a high albumin reading in an obviously thin, frail individual may be related to dehydration; the albumin level may be falsely elevated and not be truly reflective of the state of nutrition. In such cases, it becomes especially important to look at all the evidence including physical observations, other laboratory data, and the medical record. Tests and procedures can provide further insight into the patient's health. A cardiac catheterization is done in part to determine if arteries are blocked. Such a procedure should prompt the dietitian to assess lipid levels and look at other factors that may contribute to heart disease. Looking at all the data helps the dietitian determine the best course of action for each patient.

Assessment of Energy and Nutrient Requirements

Factors Affecting Energy Requirements

Energy requirements will depend on a variety of factors. Gender plays a role in energy needs because men are typically larger than women in body size; plus, muscle and fat composition are different in males and females. Men typically have greater energy needs than women. Among women, those who are pregnant and lactating have higher energy needs than those who are not. Age also plays a factor in energy needs. Given their rapid rate of growth, infants require a tremendous amount of energy for their body weight compared to an older child or adult. Adults' energy needs gradually reduce over time. Body size and composition will also affect energy requirements. Individuals with more muscle mass and overweight/obese people have greater energy requirements than someone with typical muscle mass and body size. As expected, activity level also is a factor in energy needs. A more active individual will require more energy to maintain body weight compared to someone who is sedentary. In addition, stress can have an effect on energy requirements. Someone who has undergone surgery and is healing will need additional energy to address the metabolic stress.

Calculating Energy and Nutrient Requirements

Calculating energy requirements is a normal part of the nutrition assessment. There are various methods used to calculate energy requirements, and the method should reflect the status of the individual being assessed. No method is exact, and we can only estimate needs because many factors affect the energy requirements of individuals.

Mifflin-St. Jeor:

Men: kcals/day = 10 (weight in kg) + 6.25 (height in cm) - 5 (age in years) + 5

Women: kcals/day = 10 (weight in kg) + 6.25 (height in cm) - 5 (age in years) - 161

Dietitians may also wish to use **estimated energy requirements (EERs)** to predict the energy needs of an individual. EER takes into account the age, gender, height, and activity level of the individual.

Protein needs: 0.8 g/kg/day for healthy adults.

For example, a 50 kg adult would need approximately 40 grams of protein daily (50 kg × 0.8 g/kg = 40 g).

Physical Activity Habits and Restrictions

A person's level of physical activity has an impact upon energy needs and overall health. When calculating calorie needs for an individual, the dietitian should factor in the activity level. An individual who is training for a triathlon will have different energy needs than a person who walks three times per week. In general, sedentary people require less calories in comparison to physically active individuals, but also a sedentary lifestyle may contribute to being overweight and to an increased risk of heart disease. Any activity restrictions should also be noted. Some individuals may be physically or medically unable to participate in certain activities. Someone who is wheelchair bound will have limits on physical activity, and this is an important consideration in the assessment. Someone who is elderly and has difficulty with mobility cannot achieve a high level of physical activity. There may also be medical reasons for which a person cannot participate in vigorous activity, and this is an important consideration when assessing and counseling the patient.

Comparative Standards

As the dietitian assesses and draws conclusions, it is imperative that he or she compares the data to the correct standard. There are standards for nutrients, disease states, weight, height, and laboratory test values, and it is important to reference the appropriate standard to form the correct conclusion. For example, when assessing the BMI for a 14-year-old male, the dietitian must reference the appropriate growth curve chart for a pediatric male. It would be incorrect to use the adult BMI standard for a pediatric patient. The same is true when assessing calorie and nutrient needs. The dietitian must use the appropriate standard for gender and age. Laboratory values are another standard that may vary, and it is necessary to look at the appropriate standard. The desirable A1C for a diabetic is not the same as for an individual without diabetes. Referencing the wrong standard can lead the dietitian to the wrong conclusion.

Economic/Social

Economic and social factors may provide gateways or barriers to proper nutrition. An individual with a moderate to high income has the resources to access a variety of food sources. He/she has the money to purchase foods and likely has adequate transportation to stores, restaurants, and markets. Someone living in poverty may not have adequate food dollars and/or transportation to purchase food. Housing and the ability to store and prepare foods is another consideration. Those living in poverty may have substandard housing or be homeless. A working refrigerator and stove may be unrealistic for some, and homeless persons have no shelter or reliable means to purchase and prepare food. Perhaps the individual has the financial resources, but he/she is elderly and lives alone. The individual is no longer able to drive to the grocery store and has difficulty preparing healthy meals. The dietitian must also consider one's mental wellness, any physical limitations, and alcohol/drug dependencies.

Educational Readiness Assessment

Motivational Level and Readiness to Change

The psychology of behavior change involves a number of steps; thus, behavioral change is not a quick process. Many behavioral change models exist, but essentially the steps to behavior change may be staged as follows:

1. precontemplation
2. contemplation
3. determination
4. action
5. maintenance

As a dietitian, it is important to determine at what stage the patient is in and assess their readiness to change. At the first counseling session, you may determine that the patient eats too few vegetables and fruits and is overweight. It is important to know up front where the patient falls on the readiness-to-change scale so you can tailor your message. Perhaps the initial consultation begins with precontemplation when the patient had not even considered change and ended in contemplation after the nutrition diagnoses are explained by the dietitian. Now, the patient is thinking about change, and by the next counseling session, the patient is determined to change. At this time, you can begin setting goals and having a plan of action. After change actively begins, the maintenance phase ensues, and the dietitian will continue to counsel and monitor as needed.

Educational Level and Situational

One's education level about nutrition may impact food choices, but simply understanding what is healthy does not lead to change. If one understands the importance of good nutrition and how to select healthy foods, this is one less barrier to change. A lack of nutrition education can be a roadblock for dietary change. Given the number of fad diets and opinions about nutrition circulating on the Internet, misinformation can be common. Basic education such as reading literacy may affect one's readiness and ability to change. A person's economic situation may have a tremendous impact on his or her ability to change. Although a person may have the desire to eat nutritious foods and be well-nourished, the lack of money is a barrier. Poor economic situations may lead to limited means of preparing food and an inability to afford healthy foods; a lack of transportation further exacerbates the problem. Furthermore, cultural differences can influence one's perception of eating and health. This may be further complicated if there is a language barrier. It is important to recognize cultural norms and work respectfully with the individual to bring about change.

General Wellness Assessment

A person's overall health is significant in the nutrition assessment. One's overall health may have a direct impact on his or her desire or ability to obtain proper nutrition and address dietary change. For success, it is important to look at the whole being, rather than just a single aspect of healthcare. Let us assume that our patient is paralyzed and wheelchair bound. Yes, it is important to address the nutrition diagnosis of the patient (for example, overweight), but it is essential to understand that being paralyzed affects the ability of the patient to exercise and that shopping/food preparation may be more challenging. Suppose you are assessing a diabetic patient suffering from severe depression. The diabetes is poorly controlled, and complications are a concern. It is important to understand that the patient who is severely depressed may not have the desire to control his/her diabetes. Unless the depression is addressed, nutrition interventions may be futile. The dietitian should seek to understand the patient's wellness because it may warrant a referral to another healthcare professional and could impact the nutrition care plan.

Obtain and Assess Community and Group Nutrition Status Indicators

Demographic Data

Demographic data are important because they give insight into the population being served. This information is especially helpful when conducting a community needs assessment. Information such as age, gender, race, religion, and ethnicity all play roles in the potential needs of the population being studied. Starting with age, the needs of teenagers differ greatly from the needs of the elderly. Upon conducting a needs assessment, you discover a rapidly growing aging population; this is an important finding. At this point, you must consider the services available to assist this population and pinpoint any gaps in services. Next, suppose you find a large and growing Hispanic population in the area. Cultural factors such as food preferences and choices must be considered. Furthermore, the potential language barrier should be addressed. Are there translation services available to assist in the healthcare setting? Religious beliefs may also be significant in the needs assessment. Different religions may have different dietary practices, and understanding these facts helps the dietitian tailor appropriate nutrition services. An in-depth of understanding of the community helps the dietitian address current and future needs.

Incidence and Prevalence of Nutrition-Related Status Indicators

The advantage of nutrition surveillance is that it does not provide just a single snapshot of nutrition status, but it provides ongoing information about a population. This is quite useful because populations change over time, needs change, and a continuous data stream can help pinpoint trends, either positive or negative. Many surveillance systems exist globally as well as in the United States. In the United States, the Centers for Disease Control and Prevention (CDC) is instrumental in collecting useful data about various health topics. The Behavioral Risk Factor Surveillance System (BRFSS), the National Health and Nutrition Examination Survey (NHANES), the Youth Risk Behavior

Surveillance System (YRBSS), and data from the Women, Infants, and Children (WIC) Program are all examples of surveillance programs that provide useful data for the community dietitian. Information may be gathered in a variety of ways such as data mining or with the ongoing use of surveys. A nutrition surveillance system can help identify needs; community needs will direct the actions of the community dietitian and the associated health programs. Adequate needs assessment data are essential in developing and improving community programs in the most cost-effective manner.

Prevalence of Food Insecurity

The United States Department of Agriculture (USDA) defines food security as access by all people at all times to enough food for an active, healthy life. Thus, food insecurity is a lack of access to enough food at all times to achieve an active, healthy life. To provide assistance, develop community programs, and adequately assess the patient/group, it is important for the dietitian to understand the levels of food security/insecurity of households and communities. The USDA further subdivides food insecurity into two categories:

Low food security: The diet is less optimal than desired; the quality and choice of foods may be limited, but intake appears adequate.

Very low food security: There are many issues with feeding, and intake is diminished.

Generally, very low food security results from a lack of finances. Households experiencing food insecurity report worrying about running out of food, skipping meals, hunger, and weight loss. The WIC Program and the Supplemental Nutrition Assistance Program (SNAP) are two resources aimed at bridging the nutrition gap for low-income Americans. The incidence of low food security is important when establishing nutrition programs for the community.

Reviewing and Using Nutrition Screening and Surveillance Systems

NHANES

The National Center for Health Statistics (a division of the Centers for Disease Control and Prevention [CDC]) conducts the National Health and Nutrition Examination Survey (NHANES). NHANES uses interviews and physical exams to ascertain information about health and nutritional status. The interview portion focuses on demographics plus health and nutrition status. The examination aspect of the program includes medical and laboratory data. Data uses from the NHANES survey are far reaching and include the following:

- studying the prevalence of major diseases and associated risk factors
- nutritional status as related to disease prevention
- develop standards for height and weight
- develop policy
- create new/improve existing public health programs

NHANES is a program that provides ongoing, reliable samples of data from various populations. The survey is conducted yearly and looks at a variety of health indicators. This information is very valuable as health professionals study health trends and make determinations about future needs and interventions. For example, suppose your state implemented a diabetes prevention program after determining the state's prevalence of diabetes far exceeds the national average. Measuring the success of the program would be essential, and one source of data might be information from the NHANES survey. After adequate time, you would expect the prevalence of diabetes to decrease in your state if the intervention/public health campaign is successful.

BRFSS

The Behavioral Risk Factor Surveillance System (BRFSS) is a series of health-related surveys conducted by telephone throughout the United States. The Centers for Disease Control and Prevention (CDC) originally initiated the survey, and now there are many contributing sponsors. The BRFSS provides valuable information to states about a variety of health-related topics, and some localities/metropolitan areas are now also being included in the surveys. The data collected include cholesterol awareness, fruit and vegetable consumption, and the presence of overweight/obesity and physical activity. This type of information can be useful when creating community or state awareness and intervention programs. Suppose your state initiated a campaign to get residents to eat more fruits and vegetables. The BRFSS is one source of data that could be used to measure success of the program over a number of years.

YRBSS

The Youth Risk Behavior Surveillance System (YRBSS) is conducted every two years and is aimed at collecting data for youth health risk behaviors. The YRBSS samples students in ninth through twelfth grades and monitors behaviors such as alcohol use, tobacco use, sexual behaviors, physical activity, and dietary behaviors. As with other surveillance systems, these data are important because changes in behaviors and risks can be noted over time. The community dietitian may access and use data from the YRBSS to help develop community nutrition programs targeting adolescents. The understanding that many unhealthy behaviors begin in childhood and adolescence provides an opportunity for intervention and change through education.

Importance of Considering the Availability of Community Resources

As a community dietitian, it may be necessary for you to assess the availability of community resources. This may be done as part of your community nutrition practice, or it may be conducted as part of a community nutrition program development. It is important to know what services are available for clients/patients and where there are gaps in need. For instance, if there is a large homeless population or a significant number of low-income residents, local food banks are a vital resource. Also, are there education programs aimed at the community? If the community has an increased rate of diabetes compared to the rest of the state, is there a campaign to curb these rates and improve health? It is important to understand whether basic health services are available. Do residents have easy access to a doctor and dentist? Where do the residents buy their food? Is there a grocery store nearby, or do residents have to travel a great distance to shop? Accessibility to healthcare and food may be an issue in rural areas. Often, there are barriers to success and this poses a challenge but also opens the door for program development to address those needs.

Diagnosis

Pathophysiology and Identifying Medical Diagnoses Affecting Nutrition Care

A medical diagnosis and a nutrition diagnosis are not the same. A medical diagnosis identifies the disease present, such as hypertension, cancer, or atherosclerosis. A nutrition diagnosis is identified by the dietitian and is the focus of intervention. A nutrition diagnosis might be excessive energy intake or excessive intake of saturated fat. If the diagnosis is excessive energy intake, the intervention would be to decrease energy intake (calories) by a certain amount. Of course, the medical diagnosis can impact the nutrition diagnosis. Clearly, a diagnosis of heart disease may warrant nutrition intervention, and frequently nutrition intervention can successfully improve some problems associated with heart disease.

Determining Nutrition Factors for Groups

Certain medical diagnoses and certain populations may be at risk for nutrition problems. It is important to recognize these clues during the assessment phase. Someone who has a low income or is homeless with food insecurity is at risk for malnutrition. Someone who is elderly with poor dentition, little family support, and poor ambulation may also be at risk for malnutrition. Children from low-income families who experience food insecurity may be at risk for malnutrition. Often, these children rely on school meals for nutrition because they do not receive proper meals at home. Having a certain medical diagnosis can affect one's nutrition status. For example, a diagnosis of cancer can have a detrimental effect on nutrition status. Lack of appetite and weight loss are common, and the effects of chemotherapy can exacerbate these problems. Kidney disease also has nutrition implications. Dietary intervention will be required to preserve kidney function while meeting nutrient needs.

Organizing Assessment Data and Using Standardized Language

In conjunction with the nutrition care process and outcomes focused progress, the use of standardized language and diagnosis terminology has been adopted. Dietitians use indicators or tools such as physical observation and laboratory data to determine a nutrition diagnosis. Using standardized language and a consistent approach to explain the nutrition diagnosis helps to better illustrate the rationale behind the diagnosis and planned intervention. Although many dietitians may be saying the same thing in their assessment, the information is often communicated very differently using a variety of terminology. When the terminology is consistent, it is easier to link the diagnosis, intervention, and outcomes. Healthcare interventions must be effective, and we must prove that they are effective to illustrate the necessity of nutrition intervention and to obtain payment for necessary services.

Identifying Underlying Causes and Contributing Risk Factors of Nutrition Diagnoses

Nutrition diagnosis is the second step in the nutrition care process. The nutrition diagnosis is the nutrition problem of the patient, not the medical diagnosis. The dietitian will attempt to intervene and resolve or improve the nutrition diagnosis. Critical thinking skills are important in diagnosis. He or she must consider differential diagnoses and learn to infer based on the availability of information. Nutrition diagnoses are grouped into one of three domains or categories: (1) intake, (2) clinical, and (3) behavioral-environmental. Intake can include such diagnoses as excessive energy intake or excessive carbohydrate intake. The clinical domain encompasses diagnoses such as swallowing difficulty and starvation-related malnutrition. An example of a behavioral-environmental nutrition diagnosis is undesirable food choices and food- and nutrition-related knowledge deficits. The use of standardized nutrition diagnosis terminology is an important step in furthering outcomes-based nutrition practice. Once nutrition diagnoses are identified, the dietitian should prioritize the diagnoses based on factors such as need, likelihood of success, and problem severity. Some diagnoses will require interventions that are more urgent than others.

Linking Signs and Symptoms to Etiologies

The **Nutrition Care Process (NCP)** focuses on nutrition outcomes. It is not enough to know that nutrition services are vital; in an evolving healthcare climate, we must justify the need and provide evidence. Part of illustrating the necessity of nutrition services is by linking the diagnosis, etiology, and signs/symptoms. This is done using a problem, etiology, signs, and symptoms (PES) statement. The problem is the nutrition diagnosis, etiology is something that causes or contributes to the problem, and the signs/symptoms tell us what indicators we use to diagnose the problem. For example, a PES statement for a patient showing symptoms of poorly controlled type 2 diabetes may be stated as "Inconsistent carbohydrate intake for type 2 diabetes due to lack of knowledge about dietary control as evidenced by an A1C of 8.5%." In this case, A1C is the data point that we will measure and seek to improve through dietary intervention. The problem is inconsistent carbohydrate intake, and the etiology stems from a lack of knowledge. Linking diagnosis, etiology, and signs/symptoms provides a means of showing value and effectiveness of nutrition services through the measuring of outcomes.

Documentation

SOAP Note

The **SOAP note** is one method of medical record charting that is used by dietitians and other healthcare providers. SOAP stands for subjective, objective, assessment, and plan. Subjective data include information reported to you by the patient, family, or caregivers. This might be information about feeding problems, symptoms, past medical history, food allergies, or a diet recall. The objective portion of the SOAP note details data that have been measured such as height, weight, BMI, and laboratory test values. The diet order is also included under objective data. Objective data are generally considered to be factually based information rather than reported from a patient or family member. The assessment component is where a provider draws conclusions based on the information; the assessment includes the nutrition diagnosis and level of readiness to change. Finally, the plan details the steps to address the problem, which includes goals and any planned follow-up with the dietitian.

ADIME Format

ADIME stands for assessment, diagnosis, interventions, monitoring, and evaluation, and it is a format for medical record charting. The assessment covers subjective and objective data such as reported food intolerances, diet recalls, and laboratory test value results. Diagnosis relays the nutrition problem as identified by the dietitian. As part of the Nutrition Care Process (NCP), diagnosis should be included in a PES statement. An example of a PES statement that could be included under the diagnosis is "Inadequate food intake due to poverty as evidenced by a BMI of 16.5." The PES statement details the problem, etiology, and signs/symptoms. Intervention includes planning and implementation; this is where you detail what you are going to do and how the goals will be achieved. Finally, monitoring involves tracking the progress of goals, and evaluation details the success of the intervention. This format is useful because it is in line with the NCP, and it facilitates the outcomes-based approach.

Planning and Intervention

Nutrition Intervention

Nutrition intervention is the third step in the Nutrition Care Process (NCP). As the name implies, during this phase the dietitian intervenes to address the nutrition problem. Nutrition intervention is divided into four domains: food/nutrient delivery, nutrition education, nutrition counseling, and coordination of nutrition care. The intervention phase involves planning; planning includes prioritizing diagnoses, determining outcomes, and specifying the frequency of care. Implementation of the plan also takes place during the intervention step. During implementation, the nutrition care plan is put into action.

Identification of Desired Outcomes/Actions

Evidence-Based Practice for Nutrition Intervention

As healthcare professionals trained in nutritional science, dietitians are experts in food and nutrition, and the dietetics practice applications should reflect this scientific knowledge.

Evidence-based practice recommendations compel dietetic professionals to base nutrition recommendations on scientific evidence. Research studies, surveys, and surveillance provide dietitians with a tremendous amount of useful information from which to base recommendations to individual patients or to the community. Evidence-based practice provides better outcomes for patients because the recommendations have a sound basis. Rather than making recommendations based on the latest food trend, the dietitian can look at prevalence data and see what interventions have been successful in the past. There are many health fallacies constantly circulating, but dietitians should be able to justify his/her nutrition prescription based on scientific knowledge and proven results. Evidence-based practice does not replace clinical judgement; it complements clinical judgement. The dietitian is uniquely qualified to interpret nutrition research data and apply as appropriate. In addition to improved patient outcomes, evidence-based practice offers a legitimate rationale for reimbursement from third-party healthcare payors.

Evaluation of Nutrition Information and Food Fads

Food fads come and go, and often these fads are not based on sound, scientific evidence for promoting health. Nutrition should be about nourishment and lasting health rather than the latest headline promising an unlikely or false outcome. Although some food fads do little to improve health, other food fads can actually do harm. There is an established link between what we eat/drink and our health; using a proven approach to diet rather than following ever-changing methods is advisable. A current food fad is avoidance of gluten-containing foods. Although this is necessary for those with celiac disease and those with true gluten sensitivities, there is no evidence indicating that most people should make this choice. Misinformation and the popularity of the diet leads people to avoid gluten-containing products that are generally considered healthy and a good source of fiber. Another food fad is the low-carbohydrate diet; often, this diet encourages very restrictive intake of carbohydrates while promoting higher protein foods. Such a diet becomes problematic when carbohydrates are not consumed in the balance needed and when healthy, fiber-rich foods are excluded. In addition, the promotion of protein-containing foods can result in the consumption of too much protein and unhealthy fats. Fad diets generally fail to consider a balanced approach; the dietitian is uniquely qualified to dispel food myths/fads and offer reasonable approaches to dietary health.

Health Fraud

Health fraud occurs when products claim to offer certain health benefits that are unproven and false. Often, these products sound too good to be true and offer miracle cures or astounding results.

For example, assume that there is a new plant-derived nutritional supplement on the market claiming that individuals who take the supplement will lose at least 10 pounds in 30 days. Dietetic professionals know that this claim has no merit; weight loss occurs when there is a calorie deficit, not by the action of a supplement. Individuals who desire weight loss and perhaps have been unsuccessful in the past may try this supplement. The consumer is being misled and is expecting an impossible outcome from a product with no merit. Aside from the consumer paying money for a fraudulent product, there could also be dangerous and unknown side effects. The dietitian plays a key role in educating patients, the community, and other healthcare professionals about the lack of effectiveness and potential side effects of such products.

Health and Wellness Promotion and Risk-Reduction Programs

Much like local or state health promotion programs aimed at disease prevention or reduction, employers are turning to wellness and health promotion programs to curb chronic diseases and improve health. Healthcare costs continue to increase, and a large portion of these costs may be covered by employers; it is in their best interest financially to reduce or at least contain these costs. Chronic disease can be very expensive; provider costs, hospital charges, diagnostic testing, and prescription drugs to treat the disease can be significant. There are lifestyle factors and steps that can be taken to reduce the risk of chronic disease; this has become the focus of many employee wellness programs. The program will vary depending on the company, but there are many options and many approaches. Some programs will offer screening services such as cholesterol screenings, whereas others will also incorporate smoking cessation and weight-loss programs into the mix. Employers may provide employee education in the form of a lunch and learn, whereas others offer a full healthcare clinic staffed with providers including dietitians.

Determination of Energy/Nutrient Needs Specific to Lifespan Stages

Health-Related Considerations for the Aging and Elderly

With the modern advances in medicine and technology, individuals are living longer; the result is an increasing elderly population. With age comes many physical, mental, medical, and nutrition implications that the dietitian must consider. Many nutrition-related diseases become apparent or progress as a person ages, so maintaining health and independence should be a priority for this population. With age, our bodies lose some functionality, and this is to be expected. Muscle mass tends to decrease and fat increases with age, often resulting in altered mobility. Mobility problems can affect a person's ability to shop for food and prepare meals. Physical activity can help reduce muscle loss and improve mobility. Altered taste and smell are also common with increasing age; this may result in poor dietary intake. Because taste has been affected, food may be less enjoyable. Over-seasoning of foods with salt is a potential concern, and this can be especially problematic in individuals with impaired cardiac function such as congestive heart failure. Cardiovascular decline, renal impairment, failure to thrive, and neurological changes are additional considerations for the dietitian. Each of these areas presents a unique medical nutrition therapy challenge for the dietitian.

Unique Nutrition Needs of Infants

Infants experience a rapid rate of growth compared to all other phases of life. As a rule of thumb, birth weight is typically doubled by 4–6 months of age and tripled by 12 months of age. During the first six months of life, the infant requires only breastmilk or formula. Because of the relative ease of digesting breast milk and formula compared to solids, infants eat as frequently as every 2–3 hours and are breastfed on demand. Because of the rapid rate of growth, energy and protein requirements are high compared to body weight. To promote growth and proper development, fat intake is important early in life; infants are recommended to consume at least 30 g of fat daily. The essential fatty acids arachidonic acid and docosahexaenoic acid are present in breastmilk, and formulas are supplemented with essential fatty acids. These essential fatty acids are thought to play a role in brain growth and development.

Introduction and Progression of Solids Food

Infants must develop certain skills and reach milestones prior to the inclusion of solid foods in the diet. For the first few months of life, infants have poor head control because the neck muscles are not developed. Head control, sitting up without assistance, and the ability to grasp foods are all indicators of readiness for solids. Beyond the obvious observable physical skills, oral-motor skills progress and infants are able to tolerate consistencies other than liquid. Solid food introduction typically begins at four to six months of age with cereal given by spoon mixed with a small amount of formula or breast milk. After cereals have been successfully introduced, infants may be ready to move to vegetables and fruits. Vegetables and fruits should have a puree-type consistency for ease of swallowing. In case of an allergic reaction to a new food, it is important to introduce new foods slowly and one at a time. If you were to introduce sweet potatoes, peaches, and green beans in the same day, it would be impossible to know which food caused an allergic reaction. With time, the infant will be ready for foods with more texture, finger foods, and finally table foods.

Failure to Thrive

Failure to thrive (FTT) is a growth failure defined as a weight for age below the 5th percentile on multiple occasions. FTT may also be diagnosed if weight loss falls below two growth channels on the growth chart. For example, if a child was at the 50th percentile for weight and he/she falls to below the 10th percentile, this may be indicative of FTT. Children with FTT may also have below-average head circumference, muscle wasting, and learning difficulties. FTT may result from food insecurity, medical problems, or even neglect.

Prematurity and Low Birth Weight

An infant is considered to be premature if born prior to 37 weeks' gestation. Low-birth-weight infants weight less than 5.5 lbs. Often, premature infants will also be low-birth-weight infants. Premature and low-birth-weight infants are at higher risk for poor growth and respiratory problems; other serious complications may be present depending on the gestational age of the infant. Breastmilk is especially important for preterm infants; the preterm milk differs from mature milk in that it is naturally formulated to better meet the needs of the preterm infant. The preterm infant may not suck as well as a full-term baby; if necessary, the mother can pump breastmilk to be used for enteral feeding.

Weight Gain and Energy Recommendations During Pregnancy

Energy needs during pregnancy are moderate during the first trimester but increase significantly in the second and third trimesters as the fetus growth accelerates. An additional 340 kcal/day in the second trimester and 452 kcal/day in the third trimester may be needed. Protein needs during pregnancy remain unchanged during the first 20 weeks of pregnancy, but after 20 weeks' gestation, protein needs increase to 1.1 g/kg/day. This, too, corresponds to the growing fetus. Weight gain recommendations during pregnancy vary and are dependent upon the prepregnancy BMI. In general, if the mother is underweight, a higher weight gain is desired, and if the mother is overweight, less weight gain is needed. When the prepregnancy BMI is normal, a total weight gain of 25–35 lbs is appropriate, and when the mother is underweight, 28–40 lbs should be gained. When the mother is overweight, a gain of 15–25 lbs is indicated, and with obesity, a gain of 11–20 lbs is recommended.

Nutrition for Terminally Ill Patients

Generally, end-of-life care involves comfort care measures, and therapeutic diets are generally unnecessary. The goal is to make the patient as comfortable as possible during the final time. The dietitian and healthcare team should be mindful of the patient's and family's wishes during this time. If the patient has an advance directive in place, it may indicate whether or not artificial feeding (enteral or parenteral nutrition) should be discontinued.

Steps in Nutrition Counseling

The chosen approach to counseling and education can have a tremendous influence on the information gathered by the dietitian. The receptiveness of the client/patient to intervention can also be affected depending upon the approach. Asking open-ended questions rather than yes or no questions will generally provide more and better information. For instance, you may ask, "What are some challenges you have encountered when trying to lose weight?" This question will provide better feedback than, "Are you challenged to lose weight?" Building rapport with the client is another important step. He or she needs to see that you are interested in listening, understanding, and helping rather than judging. It is important to listen, empathize, and provide feedback. Good communication can open the door to a positive working relationship with the client and may result in better client success.

Recommending Omega-3 Fatty Acids to Help Address Cognitive Function

Nutrients play a role in our physical health and our mental/cognitive well-being. Nutrients are involved in brain growth and development from the beginning of life and continue to be involved in cognitive function. The omega-3 fatty acids eicosapentaenoic acid (EPA) and docosahexaenoic acid (DHA) appear to be especially involved in brain development, function, and composition. Studies have looked at the role of omega-3 fatty acids in improving depression. Although more research is needed, some outcomes indicate improvement in depression and other psychiatric disorders when the diet is supplemented with omega-3 fats. Omega-3 fats are commonly found in fatty fish such as salmon, and consuming these fats from dietary sources is preferred. Supplementation of omega-3 fats can be used when adequate dietary intake is not possible.

Nutrient Needs of the Athlete

The nutrient needs of the athlete will vary depending on the level of activity as well as other factors such as age and gender. The needs of a high school basketball player will likely differ significantly from the needs of a swimmer training for the Olympics. Athletes who stay moderately active by exercising three times per week for about half an hour may not require a significant deviation from the norm in terms of energy requirements. Those who are active daily for approximately 90 minutes may need up to an additional 45–50 kcal/kg/day. More intensive training for longer periods of time will require additional calories, and energy needs can be quite significant. In the case of the intense physical activity and training that occurs with professional athletes and Olympic athletes, estimating energy needs can be a challenge. There tends to be a misconception about the protein needs of athletes. Your everyday, average athlete who works out three times per week may not require additional protein versus the nonathlete. Even athletes who participate in more intensive exercise generally do not require massive amounts of additional protein. As with energy intake, the protein prescription will depend on the level of activity and the type of activity, but the range is generally from 1.2 to 1.7 g/kg of body weight.

Carbohydrate Loading

Carbohydrate loading is a practice used by some endurance athletes whereby large amounts of carbohydrates are consumed in an effort to store maximum amounts of glycogen. Glycogen serves as a quick source of energy, and, in theory, increased glycogen stores should benefit the endurance athlete. Just like a car with a large fuel tank can travel farther, an athlete with more energy sources may be able to endure for longer periods of time. Carbohydrate loading works by limiting carbohydrate intake for four days followed by consuming large amounts of carbohydrates for three days prior to competition.

Implementing Care Plans

Nutrition Recommendations to Promote Wellness

The nutrition prescription is part of the nutrition care process falling under intervention. Essentially, the nutrition prescription is simply the dietitian's recommendations to the patient. The nutrition prescription should be based on a variety of factors including the nutrition assessment, nutrition diagnosis/PES statement, evidence-based practice procedures, and facility policies. The PES statement for a type 2 diabetic patient may be "Inconsistent carbohydrate intake related to lack of diabetic dietary education as evidenced by reported dietary intake patterns and A1C of 9.5%." The nutrition prescription must address the cause of the nutrition diagnosis. For our diabetic patient, the dietitian may prescribe a diet consisting of 1800 kcals daily with specific carbohydrate, protein, and fat targets. In addition, food timing and frequency may also be prescribed for the diabetic patient. Education will also be an important component of the nutrition prescription in this case because the etiology is a lack of dietary knowledge. The purpose of the nutrition prescription is to address the problem area with the goal of resolving or minimizing the issue.

Communication and Documentation

Many facilities will have interdisciplinary care teams. Care conferences are used to discuss a patient's status following clinical rounds. With this collaboration and communication, healthcare providers are able to gain additional insight into the patient's care beyond the information provided in the medical record. Interdisciplinary care teams offer many advantages, and each provider can gain insight from the unique skills of other providers. Care teams can be composed of many healthcare providers including the attending physician, nurse practitioner, registered nurses, physical therapists, social workers, psychologists, speech therapists, and the registered dietitian. Although the medical record is used to communicate pertinent information about the patient, there are limits to this type of communication, which makes the care conference very important. Take, for example, a stroke patient who was screened at admission and considered a moderate-priority patient. Upon conferencing with the speech therapist, you discover that the patient is at risk for aspiration due to swallowing difficulty that was previously unknown. Rather than wait to see this patient, he/she becomes a high priority and is seen immediately.

Identify Desired Outcomes and Actions

In order to achieve the desired objective, it is important to set measurable, realistic goals for the patient and with the patient. Goal setting is a component of intervention in the Nutrition Care Process (NCP). Goals that cannot be achieved will only produce frustration and disappointment for the patient and the dietitian. Goals that do not reflect the patient's readiness level to change will likely be set in vain. Ideally, goal setting will occur with input from the patient to help increase the likelihood of compliance. Although it might be the goal of the dietitian to see his/her diabetic patient improve A1C levels from 8.8% to 6.9%, this may not be realistic at first. Perhaps if this is the first encounter with the patient, a reasonable goal would be for the patient to improve the A1C level to 7.5% within four months. Goals should be specific, reasonable, and measurable because nutrition goals will be compared with the outcomes.

Relationship of Pathophysiology to Treatment of Nutrition-Related Disorders

Critical Care and Hypermetabolic States

Metabolic stress is multifaceted and has far-reaching implications for the body and nutrition status. Whether the metabolic stress results from injuries in a car wreck, massive burns, or surgery, the body responds in multiple ways to trauma. The body is in crisis, and all systems respond to address the threat. Glucose levels tend to rise, muscle wasting results, hormone secretion is altered, and lipid metabolism is affected. During this time, the patient may be unable to eat for a long period of time and nutrition needs may be pointedly altered based on the severity of the injury. Energy and protein needs may be significantly increased. In order to preserve lean muscle mass and adequately nourish the body to promote healing, parenteral nutrition or tube feeding may be considered. The severity of the injury and the body's response are important considerations for the dietitian as he/she prescribes appropriate medical nutrition therapy.

Eating Disorders

Anorexia Nervosa

Anorexia nervosa is essentially self-starvation with the intent to lose weight. Individuals who suffer from anorexia generally have a misperception about how their body looks while desiring to be thinner or fearing excess weight. As anorexia nervosa progresses, observable signs include extreme thinness, dry skin/hair, amenorrhea, and downy hair growth. As with other eating disorders, dietitians work with a team to successfully treat the patient. Although it is imperative, it is not enough just to restore body weight; the underlying cause of anorexia must be addressed. The treatment approach will in part be based on the severity of the anorexia. If the disease is advanced and the patient is medically comprised and extremely thin, a monitored approach to refeeding and weight gain is warranted. Eating disorder treatment programs aim to prevent further weight loss; initiate weight gain at a reasonable rate; and, finally, maintain weight. Refeeding syndrome is a concern because it can be a shock for the body to go from starvation mode to receiving nourishment. Refeeding syndrome may result in fluid and electrolyte imbalances or even cardiac arrest. A slow, monitored approach to nutrition therapy can help prevent refeeding syndrome.

Bulimia Nervosa

Bulimia nervosa is an eating disorder characterized by binge eating followed by purging. Self-induced vomiting and the misuse of laxatives are typical with these patients. Outward signs of this disorder include dental caries and sores on hands that are a result of self-induced vomiting. Unlike anorexia nervosa, patients with bulimia may be at a normal weight. The treatment for bulimia requires a multidisciplinary approach. Psychological intervention is key in treating this disorder; cognitive behavior therapy, medications, and psychotherapy may be used. The dietitian will work with the healthcare team and patient to stabilize weight and encourage positive eating practices.

Additional Eating Disorders

Because eating disorders can affect many aspects of the body, eating disorder treatment requires input from multiple healthcare professionals including physicians, psychiatrists, psychologists, and dietitians. Beyond anorexia and bulimia, several eating disorders exist. Binge eating is classified as a disorder by the American Psychiatric Association and is characterized by repeated binge eating that occurs within a specified window of time with loss of control over actions. For example, an individual with binge eating disorder may eat two boxes of cookies within 30 minutes while feeling he/she could not stop. Although most people admit to overeating at times, binge eating is recurrent, and sufferers lack the control that most people exhibit, which might otherwise prevent the behavior. Pica is another disorder characterized by the repeated ingestion of nonfood substances such as soil or ice. It is important to point out that pica may occur as a result of iron deficiency anemia rather than due to a psychiatric disorder. Rumination is the regurgitation of food and is often separate from other disorders such as anorexia and bulimia.

Food Allergies and Intolerance

Common Food Allergies and Intolerances

A food allergy results when there is an immune response to a food; the body recognizes the food as a threat or a foreign invader and elicits an inflammatory response. Food allergies often begin in childhood, but they can occur at any time; a person can be allergic to almost any type of food. The most common food allergens include peanuts, tree nuts, fish, shellfish, wheat, soy, milk, eggs, and sesame. A severe reaction to a food may result in anaphylaxis; individuals with such responses must carry injectable epinephrine in case of accidental exposure. Food intolerances differ from food allergies in that symptoms such as upset stomach are present, but there is no immune response. A common food intolerance is caused by lactose, which is found in dairy products. In lactose-intolerant individuals, the body has difficulty digesting lactose due to a lack of the lactase enzyme. Gastrointestinal upset is common with lactose intolerance, but unlike a milk allergy, a severe reaction does not occur.

Managing Food Allergies

The dietitian plays a major role in the treatment and management of food allergies. Prior to diagnosis, the dietitian may be consulted because of a suspected adverse reaction to a food. At this stage, a detailed food record indicating what is consumed, timing, and symptoms is a useful tool for the dietitian to possibly rule out a food or see a pattern. If the dietitian believes a food may be the cause of adverse reactions, this food can be eliminated from the diet for a specified period of time and then carefully reintroduced; symptoms and reactions should be noted to help determine if the food/substance is the offender. Assuming that the patient has a food allergy or allergies, the dietitian will be instrumental in educating the patient. Although someone with an allergy to tree nuts knows not to consume nuts, nuts may be unknowingly found in food products at restaurants and grocery stores. Individuals with food allergies will need to carefully read food labels, analyze menus, and speak with restaurant staff about safe choices.

Celiac Disease vs. Gluten Sensitivity

Celiac disease elicits an immune response from the body, and this response causes damage to the villi in the small intestine. Individuals with gluten sensitivity may have unpleasant gastrointestinal symptoms similar to celiac patients, but an important distinction is that there is no immune response. Although those with gluten sensitivity may experience abdominal pain and diarrhea after eating gluten-containing meals, the intestinal villi do not become damaged as with celiac disease. Because celiac disease affects the small intestines, nutrient absorption can be impaired. Anemia, osteoporosis, and other nutrient deficiencies may result. Adherence to a gluten-free diet is prescribed for those with celiac disease; this means avoiding all foods containing wheat, barley, and rye. A physician may order antibody laboratory testing for individuals suspected of having celiac disease; the presence of elevated levels of certain antibodies suggests the presence of celiac disease. Celiac disease is definitively diagnosed from an intestinal biopsy, but this is expensive and invasive.

Immune System Disorders, Infections, and Fevers

Advances in medicine now prolong and enhance the quality of life for individuals suffering from human immunodeficiency virus infection (HIV) and acquired immune deficiency syndrome (AIDS). This means that people are living longer, but it also means that there should be an increased emphasis on proper nutrition to help support the immune system and achieve or maintain a healthy weight. Because HIV/AIDS patients are living longer, they are also susceptible to chronic diseases such as heart disease and diabetes that affect the general population. HIV is a progressive disease; gradually, it attacks CD4 cells causing a compromised immune system, and it finally progresses to AIDS in which symptoms become very apparent. Once someone has progressed to AIDS, the immune system is seriously compromised. The frequency with which the patient is seen should be based on the severity of the symptoms. Antiretroviral therapy (ART) medications are used to slow the progression of HIV, and they may have side effects including diarrhea, vomiting, and insulin resistance. In addition, weight loss and other common HIV-related conditions should be evaluated by the dietitian.

Malnutrition

Malnutrition results from inadequate intake over a period of time. Generally, the longer a patient goes without meeting nutrient needs, the more malnourished/undernourished the patient will become. Weight loss, loss of muscle mass, and loss of body fat will occur and become more pronounced with time. Hospital screening tools are designed to identify patients who are malnourished and those who are at risk; malnutrition is a major concern among hospitalized patients. The approach and nutrition prescription for malnourishment will depend upon the degree of undernutrition and the medical state of the patient. A patient who is in critical care and unable to eat by mouth should be evaluated for tube feeding or parenteral nutrition. An underweight elderly patient with altered taste sensation and loss of interest in eating might warrant a different approach. If there are no contraindications to oral feeding, high-calorie supplemental nutrition options might be appropriate.

Metabolic, Endocrine, and Errors of Metabolism

Maple Syrup Urine Disease

Maple syrup urine disease is a rare metabolic disorder affecting amino acid metabolism. Leucine, isoleucine, and valine are the involved amino acids. There is a genetic link; the disease is more common in those of French-Canadian and Ashkenazi Jewish ancestry. Often, evidence of this disease will be found during newborn screening. Infants who show signs of this disorder will be lethargic, and vomiting may be present. Urine and perspiration may smell sweet. Infants with this disorder will require a special formula that omits leucine, isoleucine, and valine. This disease requires lifelong monitoring and control of amino acid concentrations. It may be possible to introduce small quantities of branched-chain amino acids into the diet if blood levels are sufficiently low.

Galactosemia

Galactosemia is an inherited metabolic disorder characterized by the body's inability to convert galactose to glucose; this occurs due to an enzyme deficiency. High levels of galactose are the result of this disorder, and this buildup causes profound complications. Infants will show signs such as lethargy, vomiting, jaundice, and failure to thrive. Early diagnosis is essential to avoid severe cognitive implications. Medical nutrition therapy is used to treat galactosemia by restricting galactose in the diet. Milk and dairy products or milk additives must be avoided. Regular infant formula and breastmilk should not be consumed; soy formula will be substituted because it does not contain galactose.

Phenylketonuria

Phenylketonuria (PKU) results from the body's inability to break down phenylalanine into tyrosine because the enzyme phenylalanine hydrolase does not function properly. The result is a buildup of phenylalanine, and this excess phenylalanine can cause brain damage. Fortunately, infants are screened at birth for this genetic condition, and although there is no cure, with treatment, serious complications can be avoided. A diet low in phenylalanine must be followed to control the symptoms of PKU. Phenylalanine is found in high-protein foods such as fish, beef, chicken, pork, and eggs; therefore, a low-protein diet must be initiated and supplemented with a special formula that provides protein. PKU is a lifelong disease and must be treated as such. Adherence to a low-phenylalanine diet helps control symptoms, prevent brain damage, and maintain quality of life.

HYPERTHYROIDISM AND HYPOTHYROIDISM

Hyperthyroidism is also known as Graves' disease and is an autoimmune disorder characterized by the overproduction of thyroid hormones. An enlarged goiter, weight loss, anxiety, and sleeplessness are common symptoms of this disorder. Medical treatment aims to reduce thyroid hormone production. When encountering the hyperthyroid patient, the dietitian should urge caution with regard to the use of supplements and botanicals because some are thought to impact thyroid activity.

Hypothyroidism results from an underactive thyroid in which not enough thyroid hormone is produced. An immune disorder, Hashimoto's disease is responsible for most cases of hypothyroidism. Hypothyroidism is treated with a replacement thyroid hormone in the form of a pill. Symptoms of hypothyroidism include intolerance to cold, dry skin, hair loss, weight gain, abnormal lipids, forgetfulness, and constipation. Vitamin D deficiency is very common in hypothyroid patients, and the patient may require supplementation. Drug/nutrient interactions may occur with the intake of synthetic thyroid hormone. Calcium-containing and high-fiber foods need to be avoided within a few hours of taking the thyroid hormone because they can interfere with absorption.

POLYCYSTIC OVARY SYNDROME

Polycystic ovarian syndrome (PCOS) involves the endocrine system and results from an imbalance in hormones. The cause is unknown, but it is fairly common and affects women of reproductive age. Symptoms include amenorrhea, dysmenorrhea, impaired glucose tolerance, hyperlipidemia, overweight/obesity, infertility, and acne. Although the name suggests the presence of cysts on the ovaries, this is not always the case. The medication commonly used to treat type 2 diabetes, metformin, is often prescribed to address insulin resistance. Hypothyroidism often presents in some cases of PCOS, and this should be investigated and treated if present. The dietitian will be instrumental in helping the patient achieve and maintain healthy weight loss if it is clinically appropriate. In addition, a low-glycemic-index diet has been shown to improve insulin sensitivity.

CUSHING'S SYNDROME

Cushing's syndrome may be characterized by the excessive presence of cortisol in the bloodstream. Although cortisol is effective in the fight-or-flight response, the presence of continuously elevated levels is harmful to the body. Cushing's syndrome may be short term in nature due to steroid medications, and it typically resolves after the medication is stopped. A more serious form of Cushing's results from a tumor on the pituitary. Weight gain and high blood pressure are common characteristics of the disease. Surgery to remove the growth is the only effective treatment. Because weight gain is common in Cushing's, weight loss counseling from the dietitian may be warranted postsurgery. For those who must remain on steroid medications long-term, the patient should be monitored for diabetes development and weight management therapy is initiated as appropriate.

ONCOLOGIC AND HEMATOLOGIC CONDITIONS

ROLE OF DIET IN CANCER PREVENTION

Cancer is not always preventable; genetic factors cannot be altered, and often environmental factors cannot be changed. Although some factors are out of our control, dietary intake is within our control, and diet plays an important role in cancer prevention. Eating adequate amounts of fruits and vegetables is an important step in overall health and cancer prevention. Antioxidants found in fruits and vegetables may play a role in cancer prevention, so it is important to eat at least five servings of fruits and vegetables daily. Red meats and processed meats should be limited because these have been linked to colon cancer, but high-fiber foods such as whole grains, vegetables, and fruits may offer benefits in preventing colon cancer. Alcohol has been linked to a number of cancers; if alcohol is consumed, intake should be limited to two drinks daily for men and one drink daily for women. Finally, overweight and obesity has been linked to some cancers, so maintaining a healthy weight should be a goal in lowering cancer risk.

Medical Nutrition Therapy Considerations

Both the cancer itself and the cancer treatment can have a profound impact on nutrition status. Cancer may affect one's appetite, and weight loss is common. As cancer advances, this scenario may become more pronounced and more difficult to manage. Side effects of chemotherapy can be severe and cause nausea, vomiting, dry mouth, altered taste/smell, and constipation. To the extent possible, the goal should be to optimize nutrition status and prevent or treat malnutrition to improve outcomes. When nausea/vomiting are present, small, bland meals should be prescribed. When a patient has little appetite, consider calorie-dense foods; small, frequent meals; and supplemental nutrition drinks to provide added calories and nutrients. Mouth sores and dry mouth caused from chemotherapy can be problematic; regular foods can be moistened with gravies or sauces; puddings, yogurt, or ice cream might be added to supplement the diet. To help relieve constipation, high-fiber foods, adequate fluid, and probiotic supplements should be encouraged. Diarrhea may result from chemotherapy, and it is important to maintain hydration by replacing lost fluids with food and drink.

Iron Deficiency Anemia

Iron deficiency anemia occurs when red blood cells do not have enough hemoglobin; hemoglobin is a protein that contains iron. To diagnose iron deficiency anemia, serum ferritin, plasma iron, and transferrin can be used; a lone measurement of hemoglobin should not be used for diagnosis. Once the diagnosis is established, iron deficiency anemia is usually treated with a ferrous iron supplement — this is the form of iron that is most readily absorbed. If possible, iron should be taken on an empty stomach for optimal absorption. If an upset stomach occurs, the supplement can be taken with food; a vitamin C-containing food/drink helps to improve absorption and should be recommended. Patients should be instructed on the dietary intake of heme iron. Heme iron is well absorbed compared to nonheme iron and is found in meat products. As with oral iron supplementation, vitamin C aids in the absorption of dietary iron sources. Inhibitors of iron absorption include fiber and tannins from coffee and tea. The patient should be instructed to avoid consuming tannins and fiber in the same meal as dietary iron sources to avoid absorption interference.

Anemias Not Related to Dietary Intake

Anemia of chronic disease is not associated with dietary intake, and individuals should not be supplemented with iron. This type of anemia is a result of disease progression and may result from cancers or infections.

Sickle cell anemia is characterized as an impaired synthesis of hemoglobin that results in sickle-shaped red blood cells. These unusually shaped red blood cells get stuck in capillaries and are not efficient at carrying oxygen. Abdominal pain may be present, which may lead to poor intake. In addition, sickle cell patients may exhibit higher metabolism rates than healthy individuals; thus, additional calories are warranted. Folate intake should be stressed, and a multivitamin containing folate, zinc, and copper may be necessary.

Pregnancy-related anemia may result from increased blood volume rather than from dietary intake. Anemia present during pregnancy should be further investigated to determine the cause or causes.

Pernicious Anemia

A lack of intrinsic factor can lead to pernicious anemia. Intrinsic factor is found in gastric acid and is necessary for the absorption of vitamin B12. Older adults are more susceptible to vitamin B12 deficiency because of a decrease in stomach acid that occurs with age. Pernicious anemia may progress slowly, but prolonged deficiency of vitamin B12 can result in nerve problems, altered coordination, and memory lapses. Because the body is unable to absorb vitamin B12, providing additional dietary sources will do little to improve the disease; instead, B12 injections are commonly given.

On occasion, vegetarians will be deficient in vitamin B12 due to a lack of dietary intake. Vegetarians should be instructed to consume foods containing B12, but other than fortified grains, vitamin B12 is generally found in animal foods. Supplementation should be considered for strict vegetarians because vegans may be unable to consume adequate amounts through dietary sources.

Organ System Dysfunction

Dysphagia

Dysphagia, or difficulty swallowing, is a common result of stroke, but it also results from other diseases including dementia, Parkinson's disease, and some cancers. Noticeable signs of dysphagia are coughing when eating and the pocketing of food. A workup by the speech therapist (ST) can provide a definitive diagnosis, and the dietitian should work closely with the ST to initiate and monitor progress of the diet. With dysphagia, the risk of aspiration exists, so swallowing and dietary progression need to be monitored. The type of diet initiated will depend on the severity of the dysphagia, but the goal is to eventually progress to a regular diet when possible. Liquids pose a risk of aspiration, so they may be thickened to help lessen this risk. The initial diet prescription for dysphagia may include pureed foods; this is the softest consistency (similar to baby food) and the easiest to swallow. The next step/progression is a mechanically altered diet, and this provides more consistency and texture. Finally, the patient may be able to advance to a mechanical soft diet. This diet includes fruits and easy-to-cut moistened meats, and it excludes dry foods and choking hazards such as nuts and popcorn. In conjunction with the ST, the diet may be progressed to a regular consistency.

Gastroesophageal Reflux Disease

Gastroesophageal reflux disease (GERD) may be present in adults and infants, and it is characterized by the reflux of stomach contents into the throat. The reflux of stomach acid can be painful and may result in more serious complications. Premature infants tend to be more susceptible to GERD, but reflux in infants typically resolves on its own with the strengthening of the sphincter muscle. Adults with GERD will likely have to deal with this chronic disease and manage the symptoms. Patients should be evaluated for overweight and obesity because these can exacerbate the symptoms of reflux. Certain foods/ingredients known as gastric irritants may aggravate symptoms; these foods include fried foods, spicy foods, caffeine, alcohol, carbonated beverages, and acidic foods. Smaller, more frequent meals as opposed to large meals three times daily may be well-tolerated and should be encouraged. Symptoms tend to be worse after eating and when lying down, so meals should conclude several hours prior to sleep.

CONSTIPATION

Constipation is characterized by difficulty in passing stools. This difficulty may make the patient feel bloated and uncomfortable. Constipation may occur as a result of disease, medications, and poor diet, but it may also occur due to an avoidance of going to the bathroom, which is common in children. A set bathroom time helps some patients retrain their bowels to promote regularity. Patients on tube feedings may experience constipation; a high-fiber formula may be necessary to help relieve the problem. Dietary intervention can help improve constipation in many cases, but for some patients, medications will also be necessary. Fluid, fiber, and activity can help promote bowel movement. Encourage patients to drink at least eight glasses of water daily and to consume whole grains, vegetables, and fruits to increase fiber intake. Fiber increases the stool's motility and softness. Physical activity can also promote bowel movement; moderate exercise should be encouraged.

PEPTIC ULCERS

Helicobacter pylori is the bacterium responsible for most peptic ulcers. Peptic ulcers can present with gastric disturbances including pain, gas, nausea, appetite loss, and vomiting. For peptic ulcers caused by H. pylori, antibiotics are typically prescribed to eradicate the bacteria. Although diet is not the cause of a peptic ulcer, dietary intervention can help manage the unpleasant symptoms associated with peptic ulcers. Gastric irritants should be avoided; spicy foods, alcohol, and caffeine may cause stomach irritation.

DUMPING SYNDROME

Dumping syndrome may occur after stomach surgery such as a gastric bypass. Rather than being digested, food moves rapidly from the stomach into the small intestine, resulting in diarrhea-like symptoms. Carbohydrates, especially simple carbohydrates such as those found in fruit juice, may make symptoms worse. This condition can generally be managed with medical nutrition therapy and will generally be short term in nature. Foods that are digested slowly such as proteins, whole grains, and fiber should be emphasized. In general, patients should avoid lactose. Smaller meals tend to be better tolerated, and it may be advantageous to avoid liquids with meals.

GAS

Gas, also known as flatulence, is a common complaint and may occur with a variety of chronic medical conditions and in healthy individuals. Gas occurs naturally and generally should not be of concern for most individuals. However, chronic conditions and certain foods may cause excessive gas and create discomfort. Medical nutrition therapy can be effective in helping to reduce excess gas. Individuals who are lactose intolerant may experience excessive gas and should avoid products containing large amounts of lactose. Patients with indigestion generally benefit from avoiding certain foods. Uncooked vegetables may increase the amount of gas produced and aggravate indigestion. Carbonated beverages and large meals may also contribute to excessive gas. If gas is a persistent problem, it may be useful to keep a food diary and note when symptoms occur to help pinpoint the food offenders.

DIARRHEA

Diarrhea may be caused by a viral infection, bacterial infection, chronic disease, or medications. The hastening of food and fluid through the bowels may result in dehydration and poor nutrient absorption. Antibiotics may cause diarrhea in some people; antibiotics attack harmful bacteria, but they also destroy useful gut bacteria. Probiotics (in supplement form or in yogurt) may be useful in combating diarrhea caused by antibiotics. When diarrhea is present, it is important to avoid further gastric irritants and ingredients that promote quick stool evacuation. Caffeine, acidic foods, and fruit juices should be avoided until the patient is well. Small, bland feedings such as crackers and toast can be initiated and should be progressed slowly as tolerated. Bananas are often well tolerated, and probiotics containing yogurt may be helpful in restoring balance to the digestive system. When diarrhea is prolonged, the patient should be monitored for dehydration and electrolyte imbalances.

Gastroenteritis

Gastroenteritis results when the stomach becomes irritated, and it may result in nausea, vomiting, diarrhea, and fever. Gastroenteritis may be caused by a contagious virus, foodborne illness, or other irritants. Typically, the symptoms will resolve within a few days, but prolonged nausea, vomiting, and diarrhea may result in dehydration and should be monitored. Parenteral nutrition may be warranted if symptoms persist. Bowel rest is appropriate with gastroenteritis; food intake can be initiated as tolerated. Lactose-containing products such as milk should be avoided because these tend to further upset the stomach. Other nonirritating liquids may be slowly introduced to help rehydrate. Solid foods may be offered; bland and dry items such as crackers and toast may be well tolerated at first. Avoid large portions and fried, greasy, and acidic foods. The patient may progress to a regular diet as symptoms subside and as tolerated.

Celiac Disease

Celiac disease is an autoimmune disorder that causes damage to the villi of the small intestine. Individuals with celiac disease have an immune response to wheat, rye, and barley. Symptoms may be difficult to distinguish from other gastrointestinal disorders, so careful investigation is warranted. Individuals may present with weight loss, diarrhea, anemia, an overall tired feeling, and bloating. A definitive diagnosis can be made with an intestinal biopsy, but often an antibody test will be used along with other information to confirm the presence of celiac disease. Lifelong strict adherence to a diet free of wheat, barley, and rye is imperative because if left untreated, celiac disease can lead to cancer, osteoporosis, and the development of other autoimmune diseases. Once treatment is initiated with diet, the villi of the intestines begin to heal and normal nutrient absorption resumes. Symptoms should begin to resolve and quality of life returns, but for some patients, even a small amount of gluten ingested can cause symptoms and can damage the villi. The dietitian is instrumental in educating the patient about foods containing gluten and some gluten-free alternatives that can be used for cooking. Generally, oats should also be avoided because of the potential for cross contamination with other gluten-containing grains. After initial diagnosis, vitamin/mineral supplementation may be warranted because of poor absorption. The dietitian should continue to monitor the celiac patient for adherence to diet, presence of symptoms, and a return to normal weight.

Diverticular Disease

Diverticula are small pouches that form in the large intestine, and when those pouches become irritated or inflamed, diverticulitis develops. Diverticulitis can cause bloating, constipation, pain, and diarrhea. Ideally, avoiding inflammation is the goal, and this may be aided by increasing fiber intake to promote intestinal motility and avoiding offending foods. When diverticulosis is present, a different dietary approach is warranted. A low-fiber, soft diet is recommended until the symptoms begin to subside. Adequate fluids may further aid in digestion, and probiotics may provide additional benefits.

Lactose Intolerance

Lactose intolerance results from the body's inability to digest lactose due to a lack of the enzyme lactase. Lactose is generally found in dairy products, so the elimination of all dairy is undesirable because dairy products do provide a good source of calcium. Often, patients who are lactose intolerant cannot tolerate milk, which is high in lactose. Milk substitutes with fortified calcium can be recommended as an alternative. Some cheeses and yogurt tend to be lower in lactose and can generally be consumed. Some examples of cheeses lower in lactose that may be well tolerated include cheddar, Parmesan, and Swiss.

Crohn's Disease and Ulcerative Colitis

Crohn's disease may occur anywhere in the gastrointestinal tract, and symptoms include diarrhea, weight loss, anemia, and cramping. **Ulcerative colitis** involves inflammation of the large intestines, and the symptoms are very similar to Crohn's disease. Given the symptoms, poor dietary intake is common and weight loss is a concern with both conditions. With Crohn's disease, inflammation is present, and the end of the small intestine is most often affected. The exact cause of Crohn's disease is unknown, but there is a genetic component to this chronic disease. Crohn's disease can have far-reaching implications including an increased risk for colon cancer, arthritis, gallstones, and bile acid malabsorption. Ulcerative colitis is also linked to genetics; the etiology is complex and not completely understood. Because digestion and absorption are significantly affected in both diseases, vitamin and mineral supplementation may be required. Specifically, calcium, folate, and vitamins D, B6, and B12 may be warranted along with omega-3 fatty acids. At times, parenteral nutrition may be necessary to achieve adequate nutrition.

Irritable Bowel Syndrome

Irritable bowel syndrome (IBS) differs from ulcerative colitis and Crohn's disease; although the symptoms may be similar, IBS does not involve chronic inflammation of the digestive system. Abdominal pain, diarrhea, constipation, and bloating are all common symptoms of IBS. The cause of IBS is not well understood, but serotonin is thought to be involved; specific testing to diagnose IBS is not available. Effective treatment can be a challenge because the cause is unknown, and stress may play a role in the worsening of symptoms. In general, treatment should be aimed at managing the symptoms. If constipation is present, fluid and fiber intake should be assessed and recommended as appropriate. Recent research suggests that limiting foods that contain fermentable oligosaccharides, disaccharides, monosaccharides, and polyols (FODMAPs) may be beneficial in the treatment of IBS.

Short Bowel Syndrome

Patients who have had bowel surgery may experience short bowel syndrome (SBS). The bowel length may be shortened due to surgery, and this compromises the ability of the bowel to absorb fluids and nutrients appropriately. The outcomes and treatment depend greatly on the amount and location of the bowel surgery/resection. Resections of the ileum may result in altered absorption of fats, fat-soluble vitamins, and vitamin B12. If the jejunum is resected, the ilium may adapt to compensate for the loss of the jejunum. Recovery can be lengthy, and it takes time for the intestines to adapt; complete resumption of normal bowel activity is unlikely in many cases. Parenteral nutrition will be initiated postoperatively, and the patient may be advanced to tube feeding while the bowel recovers and begins to adapt. Ideally, the patient will be able to progress toward an oral diet, although alternate nutrition may continue to be necessary.

Cardiovascular Disease

Cardiovascular disease, also known as heart disease, is the leading cause of death in the United States. Cardiovascular disease encompasses a variety of diseases affecting the cardiovascular system including hypertension, congestive heart failure, and atherosclerosis. Atherosclerosis involves the clogging of arteries due to fatty deposits and cholesterol called plaque. This buildup causes narrowing of the arteries and reduced blood flow. Eventually, a blockage of arteries or blood vessels may occur, and a heart attack or stroke can result. Cardiovascular disease does not begin after age 40 or age 50, but rather it is a slow, progressive process that initiates during childhood.

Although younger people do have more protection against the buildup of plaque, the disease process starts in childhood. Increasingly, high cholesterol levels have been found in children; routine screening between the ages of 9 and 11 years of age is now recommended by the American Academy of Pediatrics. This screening provides an opportunity for intervention and education that may limit or prevent the progression of cardiovascular disease for future generations.

Role of Lipids in Cardiovascular Disease

Lipids play a role in the development of atherosclerosis and heart disease. Although lipids are essential for cellular function, dyslipidemia may increase the risk for cardiovascular disease. Low density lipoproteins (LDLs) carry blood cholesterol, and high levels of LDLs are typically associated with an increased risk of cardiovascular disease. High-density lipoproteins (HDLs) are thought to help remove cholesterol; thus, higher levels of HDLs have been associated with a lower risk of heart disease. Triglycerides are fats circulating in the blood; high levels may increase the risk of heart disease.

Risk Factors for Cardiovascular Disease

Cardiovascular disease has many risk factors; some risks can be modified, but others cannot be changed. With increasing age comes an increased risk for heart disease. At age 45, men have an increased risk for heart disease; at age 55, women have an increased risk for heart disease. Overall, men are at greater risk than women of developing heart disease at any age. Hereditary factors also play a role in the development of cardiovascular disease. Some individuals may have a family history of cardiovascular disease and be genetically predisposed to adverse cardiovascular events. Age, gender, and genetics are factors that cannot be modified, but there are far more contributors to heart disease that can be altered. Overweight/obesity, smoking, lack of physical activity, excessive alcohol intake, dyslipidemia, high blood pressure, and diabetes are all risk factors that can be altered. A combination of a healthy diet, physical activity, and medication (if warranted) can help reduce the risk of cardiovascular disease.

Relevant Ranges for Blood Lipid Levels

- Total Cholesterol:
    - < 200 mg/dL is desirable.
- High-Density Lipoprotein:
    - HDL >/= 60 mg/dL is considered desirable; < 40 mg/dL is low.
- Low-Density Lipoprotein:
    - Less than 100 mg/dL is optimal.
    - 100–129 mg/dL is near optimal, but it is above the desirable range.
    - 130–159 mg/dL is considered borderline high.
    - 160–189 mg/dL is high.
    - 190 mg/dL or more is very high.
- Triglycerides:
    - <150 mg/dL is normal.
    - 150–199 mg/dL is borderline high.
    - 200–499 mg/dL is high.
    - 500 mg/dL or more is very high.

Atherosclerosis and High-LDL Management

The dietitian should assess the risk factors and attempt to address those that can be modified in order to lower LDL and prevent further plaque progression. If the patient is overweight or obese, weight reduction goals should be set. Increased weight and fat around the midsection can contribute to the development of heart disease. The diet should be low in sodium (<2,400 mg/day), alcohol intake must be moderate, and trans fats should be eliminated. Total fat should be limited to approximately 35% of total calories, and saturated fat should be limited to less than 7% of total calories. A diet high in vegetables and fruits and low in animal products should be encouraged to enhance the intake of fiber and antioxidants and decrease the intake of unhealthy fats. Healthy fats found in olive oil, fish, and nuts have shown positive effects on lipids. Plant stanols may be beneficial for some patients; food items such as margarine may have stanols added to promote heart health.

Hypertension/High Blood Pressure

Hypertension is a type of cardiovascular disease characterized by excessive pressure on the arteries and blood vessels. Hypertension is very common, it often exhibits no signs or symptoms, and the incidence increases with age. A normal blood pressure is considered to be less than 120/80 mmHg, and 130/80 mmHg or above is considered high according to the American Heart Association. Hypertension may be essential hypertension, meaning the cause is unknown, or high blood pressure may be secondary to another disease. Persistent high blood pressure can lead to heart failure, stroke, and kidney disease. Dietary intervention can have a positive effect on high blood pressure. Individuals who are overweight/obese should be advised to lose weight because increased weight is thought to be a contributing factor to hypertension. Physical activity should be recommended as another means of lowering high blood pressure. Sodium intake should be limited and alcohol consumed in moderation. The Dietary Approaches to Stop Hypertension (DASH) diet has long been prescribed and has been successful in helping to control and prevent high blood pressure. This dietary approach focuses on fruit and vegetable consumption along with consumption of lean meats, nuts, and whole grains.

Heart Failure

Heart failure, also known as congestive heart failure, is a condition characterized by the heart's inability to adequately pump blood. This weakening of the heart muscle generally occurs over time, and as the disease advances, it may result in shortness of breath, fluid retention, memory loss, and fatigue among other symptoms. Individuals with high blood pressure and a history of heart attack, diabetes, and dyslipidemia are at greater risk of developing heart failure. Patients with heart failure are frequently prescribed diuretics to rid the body of excess sodium and fluid. The nutrition prescription generally includes a low-sodium diet of less than 2,000 mg/day, fluid restrictions, weight loss if needed, a diet high in fruits and vegetables, and the DASH diet. Cardiac cachexia may accompany heart failure resulting in unintended weight loss. To help improve outcomes for cachexia, increased calories and protein may be warranted. Small, frequent meals and snacks may help provide the needed nutrients; tube feeding or parenteral nutrition should be considered if necessary.

Cystic Fibrosis

Cystic fibrosis (CF) is an incurable, inherited disease. Unlike healthy individuals with normal thin body secretions, cystic fibrosis patients have thick, sticky, and salty secretions. Although many organ systems are affected, the lungs and pancreas are the most prominent. With the increase and consistency of secretions in the lungs, chronic coughing, shortness of breath, and lung infections are quite common. Damage to the pancreas caused by the disease results in the reduced production of digestive enzymes. Without adequate digestive enzymes, fat malabsorption and absorption of fat-soluble vitamins become impaired. Physicians will typically prescribe pancreatic enzyme replacement therapy to help with nutrient absorption. CF may also lead to pancreatitis, diabetes, and bone disease. Patients with CF are prone to growth failure because of increased energy needs and poor absorption. Increased calorie intake and supplementation of fat-soluble vitamins are necessary; in addition, liberal sodium intake may be encouraged to replace losses in secretions. Depending on secondary problems, additional dietary intervention may be warranted to address pancreatitis and diabetes.

Chronic Obstructive Pulmonary Disease

Chronic obstructive pulmonary disease (COPD) is a lung disease that involves impaired airway flow and includes conditions such as chronic bronchitis and emphysema. Shortness of breath and coughing are typical with COPD. Weight loss is common in COPD patients, and this may lead to poor outcomes. Due to the effects of the disease and difficulty breathing, the COPD patient will burn more calories than a healthy individual. If the patient is malnourished, increased calories and protein are prescribed. Achieving and maintaining a healthy weight should be a primary goal of the nutrition plan. Limited sodium intake, small frequent meals, and adequate intake of essential fatty acids should be encouraged.

Liver

The liver is an essential organ involved in the metabolism of carbohydrates, fats, and protein. The functions of the liver are complex; beyond metabolism, the liver also filters and detoxifies. Bile production takes place in the liver; bile helps break down fats for use as energy or for storage. The liver produces cholesterol and removes cholesterol from the bloodstream. The liver also serves as the storage area for fat-soluble vitamins and plays a role in the regulation of carbohydrates. When blood glucose levels fall too low, the body breaks down glycogen; glycogen is the stored form of glucose. When blood glucose levels are too high, the liver will store the glucose for later use. Glucose-6-phosphatase is a key enzyme involved in regulating glucose concentrations.

Medical Nutrition Therapy for Cirrhosis

Liver cirrhosis is a progressive disease characterized by damage to the liver caused by a variety of factors including alcoholism, viral hepatitis, and cystic fibrosis. Once liver function is lost, it cannot be restored. The goal is to slow and control the disease to the extent possible. Ascites is a common result of cirrhosis. Ascites occurs because of a chain of events; the damaged liver has impaired blood flow, causing portal hypertension. Portal hypertension results in the kidney's inability to properly remove fluid and electrolytes. A noticeable sign of ascites is abdominal edema. Sodium intake should be limited to 2 g/day, and fluid intake should be restricted when ascites is present. Alcohol should be eliminated from the diet, especially when alcohol is the cause of the cirrhosis. The liver filters alcohol, and the by-product of alcohol metabolism is detrimental in large quantities. Adequate protein, additional calories, and essential fatty acids may be prescribed.

Medical Nutrition Therapy for Hepatitis

Hepatitis is an inflammation of the liver and may result from a virus or toxicity. Those affected by hepatitis will typically be jaundiced with nausea and vomiting present. Viral hepatitis can be transmitted from person to person. Hepatitis A can be passed on through contaminated food and drinking water; poor food handling practices and unsanitary conditions are generally to blame. Medical nutrition therapy for hepatitis includes a higher intake of protein than normal at 1–1.2 g/kg/body weight. Protein has been shown to prevent a fatty liver. Calorie needs may also be above average at 30–35 kcal/kg body weight.

Gallbladder Disease

The gallbladder stores bile; bile is essential in the digestion of fats. Cholelithiasis is the term used to indicate that gallstones are present in the patient. Cholecystitis is an inflammation of the gallbladder. Removal of the gallbladder is a common treatment for troublesome cholecystitis with cholelithiasis present. Patients who have had their gallbladder removed will initially be on a low-fat diet but may progress to a regular diet. Patients with acute cholecystitis benefit from no oral intake, and parenteral nutrition should be initiated if intake cannot be resumed within a reasonable length of time. Chronic cholecystitis patients benefit from ongoing low-fat diets; high-fat diets have been linked to gallstone production, whereas plant-based diets may inhibit the production of gallstones.

Acute and Chronic Pancreatitis

Pancreatitis is a painful inflammation of the pancreas. The pancreas aids in digestion and produces insulin. Acute pancreatitis is generally short-term in nature and may be treated with medical nutrition therapy by discontinuing oral feedings and providing fluids intravenously. Tube feeding should be considered when oral feeding cannot resume within a reasonable amount of time. Oral intake should progress slowly with small, frequent meals that are low in fat. Chronic pancreatitis is a long-term problem. Significant problems that may result in malnutrition with chronic pancreatitis include pain associated with eating, nausea, and vomiting. Small, frequent low-fat meals should be prescribed. Although oils and fats should be limited, medium-chain triglyceride (MCT) oil may be beneficial due to the altered fat absorption occurring in pancreatitis.

Type 1 Diabetes and the Associated Nutrition Intervention

Type 1 diabetes is an autoimmune disease in which the body attacks the beta cells of the pancreas. Eventually, the body will lose its ability to produce insulin and lifelong insulin replacement is necessary. Type 1 diabetes has an early onset, and the specific cause is unknown, but there is a genetic component. Unlike type 2 diabetes, type 1 diabetes is not preventable. Symptoms of type 1 diabetes include weight loss, frequent urination, increased thirst, and fatigue. Diabetic complications are numerous, so controlling blood glucose and limiting risk factors for heart disease are essential in the prevention of secondary problems. Patients may use injectable insulin needles or an insulin pump. Monitoring of blood sugar levels with finger sticks is essential in properly regulating diet and insulin dosage. The patient should be instructed on carbohydrate counting, and a meal plan should be based on individual needs. Because cardiac complications are a common result of diabetes, the diet should be heart healthy with a limited intake of saturated fats and trans fats.

Type 2 Diabetes

Type 2 diabetes is a result of the body's inability to properly use insulin. Unlike type 1 diabetes, the body still produces insulin, but gradually insulin production will decrease. Type 2 diabetes typically has a later onset than type 1 diabetes, although type 2 diabetes is being diagnosed in younger patients due to poor dietary and exercise habits. Type 2 diabetes is largely preventable; positive lifestyle choices can help reduce the risk of developing type 2 diabetes. Individuals who are overweight or obese are more likely to develop type 2 diabetes, so maintaining a healthy weight is important. Lack of physical activity, abdominal fat distribution, and family history also play a role in the development of type 2 diabetes. Symptoms include frequent urination, increased thirst, hunger, and blurred vision. With type 2 diabetes, it is important to control blood sugar and try to prevent secondary complications of diabetes such as heart disease and kidney disease.

Diagnostic Criteria

The following labs are indicative of the presence of diabetes:

A1C: 6.5% or higher (normal is 4-5.6%).

Fasting Plasma Glucose: 126 mg/dL or higher (normal is 99 mg/dL or less).

Oral Glucose Tolerance Test: 200 mg/dL or higher (normal is 139 mg/dL or less).

If test results indicate diabetes, a second test should be performed to confirm the diagnosis.

Prediabetes Diagnosis

Individuals who have a fasting glucose between 100 and 125 mg/dL or a higher than normal A1C may be classified as having prediabetes. Individuals with prediabetes are very likely to develop type 2 diabetes, but once prediabetes is detected, lifestyle changes can help alter the outcome. Often, weight loss is needed; weight reduction can help reduce the risk of progression to type 2 diabetes. Dietary modifications including calorie reduction, an emphasis on fruits, vegetables, and whole grains combined with intake of healthy fats can improve overall dietary health. A physical activity program should be encouraged to help with weight loss and improved glucose control.

Medical Nutrition Therapy for Type 2 Diabetes

It is important to normalize blood glucose levels as much as possible. A1C goal levels should be less than 7%, and fasting blood glucose should be between 90 and 130 mg/dL, whereas postprandial levels should remain less than 180 mg/dL. To properly address type 2 diabetes, weight loss in many patients will be necessary. Weight loss has been shown to have a positive effect on blood sugar levels and lipid levels. Meal plans will be individualized based on needs, but carbohydrate intake ranges from 45%–65% of total daily calories. Protein recommendations should be 15%–20% of total calories, and fat makes up 25%–35% of total calories. A diet high in plant-based foods and low in saturated fats and animal products should be encouraged. A major risk factor for heart disease is the presence of diabetes, so dietary approaches to help prevent heart disease are important to emphasize. The patient should be educated about the importance of regular mealtimes, consistent carbohydrate intake, lipid management, and physical activity.

Common Medications Used for the Treatment of Type 2 Diabetes

Although the initial treatments for type 2 diabetes include diet and lifestyle modification, some individuals who are not meeting blood glucose goals will need medication therapy. There are a variety of medications used to treat type 2 diabetes. Metformin, classified as a biguanide, is one of the most commonly used drugs to treat diabetes. Metformin works on the liver to decrease the amount of glucose made. Sulfonylureas and meglitinides both work on the pancreas, causing a release of more insulin. Thiazolidinediones improve the efficiency of insulin and decrease glucose production. Sulfonylureas and thiazolidinediones may cause weight gain, whereas metformin has been associated with modest weight loss. Type 2 diabetics who can no longer produce enough insulin will need injectable insulin to properly control blood glucose to minimize diabetic complications.

Gestational Diabetes

Gestational diabetes occurs during pregnancy and typically goes away shortly after birth. Although gestational diabetes is a short-term condition, it does put the patient at risk for developing type 2 diabetes later in life. Gestational diabetes can increase the risk of having a large-for-gestational-age baby, and other complications may arise. A meal plan should be established that provides adequate carbohydrates and nutrients but limits excess carbohydrates that may increase blood glucose levels beyond what is desired. It is important to focus on adequate weight gain and limit excessive weight gain during pregnancy. The dietitian should encourage physical activity, intake of adequate calories to meet the needs of pregnancy, and healthy intake including whole grains and limited sweets.

Insulin

Several types of insulin are available, and they can be prescribed for type 1 diabetes and if warranted, type 2 diabetics whose insulin production has diminished significantly. Insulin may be categorized as long acting, intermediate acting, short acting, and rapid acting, referring to the length of time between the injection and when the insulin begins to work. Rapid-acting insulin begins to work most quickly, and long-acting insulin begins to work within two to four hours of injection; long-acting insulin may be effective for up to 24 hours. A bolus injection of insulin is typically given prior to meals to help counteract the typical peak in glucose levels that occur postprandial. The bolus injection works quickly, and the amount of bolus insulin is adjusted based on the carbohydrates consumed. For many, the insulin pump has provided freedom from the typical regimen of needles and injections. The pump is programmed to deliver a constant flow of insulin into the body, and bolus doses may be given to cover meal carbohydrate intake.

Carbohydrate Counting in the Management of Diabetes

Carbohydrate counting is an essential aspect of diabetes management because carbohydrates, although necessary, affect blood glucose levels. When inadequate or no insulin is present in the blood, blood glucose levels remain high. Having a meal plan that involves carbohydrate counting helps individuals who are not dependent on insulin limit excess carbohydrates. For individuals who are on an insulin regimen, carbohydrate counting is essential for overall control and is useful for calculating bolus injections. Carbohydrate counting also provides flexibility with meal plans; individuals can substitute one serving of carbohydrate for another. When counting carbohydrates and exchanging foods, approximately 15 g of carbohydrates are considered to be one serving. This means that an individual can replace a slice of bread with a piece of fruit and the total carbohydrate count remains basically the same. When setting up a meal plan, the dietitian will recommend a certain number of carbohydrate servings per meal/snack, and the patient has flexibility in choices.

Carbohydrate Exchange List

Food Group	Carbohydrates (g)	Protein (g)	Fat (g)	Calories
Starches/ grains, starchy vegetables, beans	15	3	1	80
Fruit	15	0	0	60
Skim 1% milk	12	8	0–3	90
Reduced-fat milk 2%	12	8	5	120
Whole milk	12	8	8	150
Nonstarchy vegetables	5	2	0	25
Lean protein	0	7	2	45
Medium-fat protein	0	7	5	75
High-fat protein	0	7	8	100

Complications Associated with Diabetes Mellitus

Long-term complications from diabetes are many; this is why it is so important to control blood glucose helping to minimize the risk of developing secondary problems. Diabetes is a risk factor for heart disease. Dyslipidemia often accompanies diabetes, and this combined with the cardiovascular damage caused by diabetes puts the diabetic at significant risk. In addition, hypertension is often present in diabetes, further increasing the risk. It is imperative that while addressing blood glucose control, a heart-healthy approach to diet and activity also be implemented. Diabetic nephropathy (kidney disease) and diabetic retinopathy (eye disease) are also frequent compilations of diabetes. Nerve damage known as neuropathy is very common among diabetics; in very serious cases of uncontrolled diabetes and neuropathy, limb amputation can result. In the short term, diabetics often experience hypoglycemia, or low blood sugar. Diabetic ketoacidosis (DKA) may result when there is a lack of insulin. DKA is very serious and may result in death if not treated.

Renal System

The kidneys are complex, multifaceted organs. The renal system works as the body's waste filter and is responsible for maintaining homeostasis. The kidney is responsible for regulating electrolytes and maintaining proper fluid balance; it also plays a role in the regulation of blood pressure. The renin angiotensin system helps to maintain adequate blood pressure by converting angiotensin to angiotensin II. In addition to filtering and regulation of blood pressure, the kidney produces erythropoietin, which is involved in the production of red blood cells. D-1,25-dihydroxycholecalciferol (the active form of vitamin D) is also produced in the kidneys.

Medical Nutrition Therapy for Kidney Stones

Kidney stones are painful stones generally made up of calcium. Individuals who experience kidney stones may benefit from weight loss if the BMI exceeds 25. For individuals with stones consisting of calcium, dietary intake of calcium is actually associated with a lower risk of stone formation. Calcium supplementation does not appear to have the beneficial effects of dietary calcium. A higher rate of stone formation has been found in individuals taking calcium supplements. Although dietary intake of calcium is preferred, those who cannot consume adequate dietary calcium may choose supplementation. Taking calcium supplements with meals is recommended; supplementation with meals may help to counteract the negative effects that calcium supplementation can have on calcium stone formation. A diet limiting excessive amounts of oxalate may also be warranted to combat stone formation. Foods high in oxalate include spinach, rice bran, corn grits, French fries, cocoa powder, and raspberries.

Acute Renal Failure vs. Chronic Renal Failure

Acute renal failure is also known as acute renal injury; it is a reduction in the kidney's filtration rate. Acute renal failure may require short-term dialysis until the condition resolves. Acute renal injury is temporary in nature, whereas chronic renal failure is a permanent, progressive disease. Patients with chronic renal failure have many health implications, and preserving renal function for as long as possible is important. Uncontrolled diabetes and hypertension are two major causes of chronic renal failure. Eventually, end-stage renal disease (ESRD) may result from chronic renal failure. When the body is no longer able to efficiently filter waste products, the course of treatment is dialysis or kidney transplantation. Hemodialysis and peritoneal dialysis are two distinct dialysis options for patients; ongoing dialysis treatment may take place in an outpatient facility or at home with special dialysis equipment.

Chronic Kidney Disease

With chronic disease, the goal is to preserve kidney function and put off dialysis for as long as possible. Chronic kidney disease is progressive and is staged according to the degree of insufficiency. Stage 1 is the earliest stage and shows normal filtration rates. Stage 2 begins to show impaired filtration rates, but it is likely to go unnoticed without laboratory testing. Further decreases in the glomerular filtration rate occur as the disease progresses and symptoms become apparent. Stage 5 is the final stage and is known as end stage renal disease (ESRD). Dietary modification will be individualized and is based largely upon disease staging. Sodium and processed food intake should be modest. Protein intake for stages 1–3 is within the normal range of 0.8–1.0 g protein/kg of body weight per day. Protein is reduced when the patient enters stage 4 to 10% of calories per day. For example, a patient on a 2,000-calorie diet would be prescribed 50 g of protein/day. 2,000 kcals × 0.10 = 200 kcals/4 kcals/g = 50 g.

End-Stage Renal Disease

At the point of end-stage renal disease (ESRD), the patient must begin dialysis in order to survive. To some degree, the diet can be liberalized because of mechanical filtering of the blood. The nutrition prescription will vary somewhat depending on the type of dialysis. As always, it is important to optimize the diet and treat or prevent malnutrition. Calcium and phosphorus are not adequately removed through the process of dialysis, so intake must be limited to maintain proper balance. Calcium intake should be less than 2,000 mg/day, and phosphorus intake should be limited to 800–1,200 mg/day. Individual fluid recommendations should be based on fluid output and hydration status. The protein requirement for hemodialysis are approximately 1.2 g/kg/day. It may be slightly higher for peritoneal dialysis patients at 1.2–1.3 g/kg/day. Because peritoneal dialysis occurs daily, more potassium is lost in the process; increased potassium is typically prescribed.

Orthopedic/Wounds

Metabolic Stress

The body responds to metabolic stress through a variety of mechanisms. Whether the metabolic stress is caused by major burns, sepsis, surgery, or a catastrophic accident causing wounds, the body may go into a state of shock. The body will likely begin by breaking down muscle, decreasing blood flow, and decreasing insulin production. After this initial shock response, the body will begin to normalize cardiac output, glucose production increases, and the hormones glucagon and cortisol are released. Glucagon signals for an increased production of glucose. Critical patients will frequently have very high levels of blood glucose; under these circumstances, you should not assume that diabetes is present unless it has been previously diagnosed. In addition, lipid levels may be unusually high. Cortisol is released during stress and is involved in the fight-or-flight response. Cortisol released in small doses is beneficial, but prolonged high levels of cortisol during stress can have unwanted effects.

Wound Healing

Third-degree burns are the most severe and cause major damage to body tissues. Special burn units are available to treat patients who have experienced severe burns. A burn patient may be under a great deal of metabolic stress, and this stress may be prolonged throughout the recovery period. The exact approach to treatment will depend on the total body surface area burned and the depth of the burn. Burn patients lose a tremendous amount of fluid, so the initial step in medical nutrition therapy is to replace fluids. Enteral nutrition should be initiated, and it has been shown to improve outcomes in burn patients. Calories will vary depending on the surface area and depth of the burn, but energy needs are expected to be significant compared to a healthy individual. Protein needs will also be increased to approximately 1.5 to 3.0 g/kg of body weight. Supplemental vitamin C and zinc sulfate should be considered to help with wound healing.

Osteoporosis and Osteopenia

During the early years of life, one's bones build bone mass. In the later years, bone mass is gradually lost. After menopause, the rate of bone loss in women becomes more evident because of a lack of estrogen. Although men lose bone mass with age, the loss is less significant compared to women. Osteopenia is characterized by less-than-normal bone mass; osteopenia is less severe than osteoporosis. Osteoporosis is significant loss of bone mass that results in fragile bones. Risk factors for decreased bone mass include age, female gender, excessive alcohol intake, smoking, ethnicity, small frame/low body weight, and inactivity. To promote bone density, physical activity and strengthening exercises should be encouraged. Calcium and vitamin D intake should be optimized. Dietary sources of calcium are best absorbed and should be encouraged instead of supplementation. Supplementation is acceptable when individuals are unable to meet their needs through diet.

Obesity

Overweight and Obesity

The issue of overweight and obesity has become an enormous problem in the United States. Many health problems are secondary to increased weight, and the rise in these chronic diseases puts a strain on our healthcare system and affects quality of life. Factors such as a lack of physical activity, poor dietary intake, and genetics contribute to overweight and obesity. In adults, a BMI of 25 or above is considered overweight, whereas a BMI or 30 or greater is indicative of obesity. The patient's state of overweight and obesity is determined using a growth chart for children and teens. The approach to treating overweight and obesity should focus on long-term achievement and maintenance of a healthy weight. Frequently, weight lost will be quickly regained when the "diet" is abandoned. Depending on the BMI, a weight loss of 1/2 pound to 2 pounds per week is considered desirable. Dietitians may prescribe a reduced calorie diet with physical activity to help promote weight loss. The success of weight loss and maintenance depends on the patient's willingness to embrace lifestyle changes.

Obesity Management in Adults

When implementing a weight loss program, the dietitian must assess the patient's readiness to change. A great deal of responsibility on the part of the patient will be required to be successful in weight loss and weight maintenance. A well-balanced meal plan should be prescribed that includes a reduction in calories. High-fiber foods should be encouraged because of the health benefits and because of the slower rate of digestion. High-fiber foods may help the patient feel full longer. In addition, healthy fats and lean proteins should be stressed. Fats and proteins are digested more slowly than carbohydrates and may help with satiety. Lean protein choices include fish, poultry, and low-fat dairy. Healthy fats such as olive oil can be used for cooking. A carbohydrate-restricted diet is not recommended; rather, a carbohydrate intake of 35%–50% of total calories is recommended. Whole grains should make up a significant portion of the total carbohydrate intake. Adults should keep a food journal and weigh frequently to assess their progress. The dietitian is instrumental in providing education and support and in adjusting the nutrition prescription as needed.

Alternative Treatments for Obesity Management in Adults

Many approaches to weight loss have been suggested over the years. Although people want a quick and easy approach, fad diets and supplements are often ineffective and unsafe. Very-low-calorie diets consist of fewer than 800 calories daily. Such severe calorie restrictions cannot be maintained long term, and although weight loss does occur, weight loss is unlikely to be maintained over a longer period of time. Prescription weight loss medications may be initiated to supplement dietary intervention and improve weight loss outcomes. Such medications work by acting on the brain or in the case of orlistat, fat absorption is decreased. Bariatric surgery may be used in the morbidly obese individual (BMI at or above 40) or in individuals with a BMI of 35 or greater in the presence of another condition such as diabetes. Bariatric surgery should not be considered unless other interventions have failed.

Obesity Management in Children and Adolescents

Obesity has become a significant problem in youth, and although intervention programs are aimed at reducing the rates of overweight and obesity, the problem persists. Weight management in this group may be handled differently than weight loss in adults. Because young people are still in the growth phase, a different approach is often warranted. As with adults, encouragement of healthy eating habits and physical activity is encouraged. Parental involvement is important in this step because often children do not make their own meal choices. For younger children who have a BMI at or above the 85th percentile, slowing the rate of growth is preferable. When weight gain slows, the child will continue to grow taller and BMI will become normalized. If the child has a BMI at or above the 95th percentile with a complicating factor such as hypertension, weight loss may be necessary. For older children, with a BMI at or above the 85th percentile, weight maintenance should be encouraged. When complications such as hypertension or hyperlipidemia are present, or the BMI is at or above the 95th percentile, weight loss is typically prescribed.

Cleft Lip and Palate

A cleft lip is a birth defect in which an opening in the lip is present; there may be an opening on only one side or on both sides of the lip. A cleft palate is characterized by an opening in the roof of the mouth. Surgery is required to correct these conditions, and often multiple surgeries/repairs will need to occur depending on the severity. Although there appears to be no one cause for these birth defects, one risk factor is a lack of maternal folic acid. Feeding is generally affected because the lips and oral cavity are not properly formed. Infants typically have difficulty breastfeeding because of poor sucking ability. It may be necessary for the mother to pump breastmilk or use formula. When bottle feeding, special adaptive bottles and nipples that reduce the need for sucking may improve feeding. If the infant is unable to meet needs with a regular infant formula, a higher calorie formula may be appropriate.

Prader-Willi Syndrome

Prader-Willi syndrome is a chromosomal disorder that tends to cause extremes in appetite leading to increased weight and obesity. Developmental delays and short stature are also common characteristics. Short stature has been linked to a deficiency in growth hormone, and it may be treated with replacement hormone therapy. A lack of control when eating and insatiable appetite may be caused by a disruption in the hunger-satiety feedback mechanism of the hypothalamus. Controlling weight is of primary importance in these patients, and this is made difficult given the lack of satiety and decreased metabolic rate. Excessive weight gain is very common. Young children need to be given set meal times and snacks, or continuous intake may occur leading to rapid increases in weight. As the child ages, specific caloric intake should be recommended, and it may be necessary to provide physical barriers to food such as locking cabinets and refrigerators. Weight management protocols and encouragement of physical activity will need to continue throughout the lifespan.

Cerebral Palsy

Cerebral palsy (CP) is caused by a brain injury in utero or during infancy. CP-associated problems result from difficulty in muscle control due to the brain injury, and the severity varies. The most severe and complex forms of CP can result in quadriplegia, but, in general, difficulty with movement, involuntary movements, and muscle tone abnormalities are common. In addition, cognitive function may be affected, but this is not always the case. The dietitian should be concerned with feeding difficulties causing inadequate growth and constipation. Obtaining a correct height may be difficult given muscle contractures and an altered ability to stand/walk. Estimates using the arm span and lower leg length may be appropriate. Because of the multitude of problems present in more severe cases, achieving adequate nutrient intake can be difficult. Tube feeding may be required to achieve adequate nutrient and energy intake.

Feeding Difficulties Encountered in Autism

Autism is considered to be a neurologic disorder, and it includes Asperger syndrome. Autism is characterized by limited social abilities, and speech may be delayed. The exact cause of autism is unknown, but environmental and genetic factors are thought to be involved. Cognitive abilities may be compromised in autism, but those with Asperger syndrome typically exhibit normal intellectual abilities. From a dietary standpoint, food and texture aversions are common concerns; it may be necessary to work with a speech therapist to address these issues. The feeding abilities of some infants and children may progress well and on schedule, whereas others will have delays; the interventions will depend on the problems presented. Some individuals with autism will benefit from eating in a quiet, non-hectic environment. If the child is underweight, high-calorie snacks can be offered. The parent should be counseled on how to deal with texture aversion and food jags.

Down Syndrome

Down syndrome results from the presence of an extra chromosome (47 chromosomes rather than 46). Patients with Down syndrome have cognitive impairment and may also present with congenital heart disease, delayed growth, overweight, dental problems, and hypothyroidism. When assessing the patient with Down syndrome, it is important to understand that because of short stature, the BMI will be higher than for a healthy individual; the BMI should not be compared to the reference standard for healthy individuals. Physical delays such as poor head control may necessitate the need to delay solid food introduction during infancy. Overall, feeding progression is likely to be slower than in a healthy infant/toddler. Adequate calories and nutrients should be prescribed to meet needs, but overfeeding and overeating should be discouraged. Overweight is a problem in Down syndrome, so encouraging physical activity and regular meal/snack times is important. Discouraging the use of sweets, fast food, and sugary drinks may help to limit excess weight gain.

Kwashiorkor and Marasmus

Kwashiorkor and marasmus are extremes in pediatric protein-energy malnutrition. These conditions often occur together and are very serious. Rarely are these conditions seen in the United States, but children in developing countries may be affected due to starvation. Those affected by kwashiorkor will be very thin, appear frail, exhibit loss of muscle mass, and may have a large, distended abdomen filled with fluid. Children with marasmus look emaciated and may appear listless. These conditions can cause permanently altered growth, affect cognitive development, and result in death if the malnutrition is not corrected in a timely manner.

Preeclampsia

Some pregnant women may experience an increase in blood pressure during the second half of pregnancy. In some cases, no further complications arise, but for some women, preeclampsia results. Generally, those with preeclampsia will have increased blood pressure and protein in the urine (proteinuria). Preeclampsia is a high-risk condition and can be life-threatening for the mother and fetus. When diagnosed with preeclampsia, patients may be confined to bed rest. Babies are often premature because labor may need to be induced to prevent further complications or death. A maternal diet adequate in calories, calcium, folic acid, potassium, and magnesium is recommended.

Mediterranean Diet

The Mediterranean diet is not really a particular diet; rather, it is a way of eating similar to the dietary patterns seen in the Mediterranean Region of Europe. Why would we recommend emulating those patterns? When this region's diet was first studied after World War II, the results were surprising to many. These populations were found to have a much lower incidence of diabetes, heart disease, and cancers. Plus, they were living longer than residents of the United States and many other developed countries. When studying their dietary patterns, it was clear that this population consumed mostly a plant-based diet. Meats/proteins were consumed on occasion, and the meat usually consisted of fish. The majority of their fat intake came from consumption of olives and olive oil. A diet derived mostly from plants with limited intake of saturated fats, a higher proportion of omega-3 fats, and limited protein was found to be superior when compared to the typical American diet. Dietitians know that this approach is a healthful one, so it is a dietary approach that is often recommended to treat the symptoms of cardiovascular disease or simply as a healthy approach to eating.

Metabolic Syndrome

Metabolic syndrome is characterized by the presence of multiple symptoms (three or more) such as hyperglycemia, obesity/high waist circumference, hypertension, and dyslipidemia. Because metabolic syndrome indicates the presence of multiple risk factors, having metabolic syndrome greatly increases the chance of developing cardiovascular disease and diabetes. Interventions include weight loss, physical activity, the Mediterranean diet, the DASH diet, and a controlled carbohydrate intake.

Pressure Ulcers

Pressure ulcers are also known as bed sores and are common among bedridden patients such as those found in long-term-care facilities. Malnutrition and lack of mobility may contribute to the development of pressure ulcers. Pressure ulcers are staged based on severity. Stage I involves intact skin, but redness may be present. Stage II presents as a more obvious sore but involves only the skin surface. Stage III is more pronounced with a full loss of tissue. Stage IV is extreme and exposes open areas below the tissue such as bone and muscle. Adequate nutrition is important in addressing pressure ulcers, but alone nutrition will not heal the condition. Proper nutrition along with correct wound dressing and repositioning can help in managing the pressure ulcer. The dietitian should recommend a protein intake of 1.25–1.5 g/kg/day; protein supplements may be necessary to achieve this goal. The patient may benefit from a multivitamin; vitamins and minerals important in wound healing include zinc, copper, and vitamin C.

Hypoglycemia

Hypoglycemia occurs when blood glucose levels fall below 70 mg/dL. Type 1 diabetics who have injected too much insulin may suffer from hypoglycemia, and it may also occur in type 2 diabetics due to medication. Glucose tablets or 4 oz. of fruit juice may be used to counteract episodes of hypoglycemia by providing quick sources of glucose. Educating the diabetic patient is an important step in preventing hypoglycemic episodes. The dietitian should stress regular blood glucose monitoring and consistently adhering to meal plans.

Gout

Gout often causes painful arthritis resulting from a buildup of uric acid. Excess uric acid is present due to a metabolic disorder that is thought to have a hereditary component. Gout can be a long-term problem with recurrent episodes; medications may need to be prescribed that lower uric acid levels. Dietitians should recommend avoiding alcohol and fructose because these may increase urate production. A low-fat, low-carbohydrate diet may help with ridding the body of urates.

Urinary Tract Infection

A urinary tract infection (UTI) is caused by a bacterium and results in painful urination. Because of their anatomical makeup, women are more likely to get UTIs than men. If left untreated, a UTI can affect kidney function. Antibiotics are typically prescribed to treat the infection, and drinking cranberry juice has long been recommended in helping resolve UTIs. Cranberry juice is thought to provide an acidic environment inhibiting the growth of bacteria. Fluid intake should be liberal, and caffeine, a diuretic, should be avoided.

Varying Energy Needs

Energy needs will vary greatly depending on factors such as age, gender, current weight/height, and medical diagnosis. Patients who are experiencing metabolic stress resulting from surgery, burns, or other wounds generally require significantly more calories and protein than a healthy individual. Patients who are overweight and obese require more calories than a normal-weight individual to maintain weight, but calorie restrictions are prescribed to promote weight loss. Patients with COPD have difficulty breathing, and this extra breathing effort increases energy needs. Patients will renal failure typically should be prescribed less protein than healthy individuals to help preserve kidney function. There is not a "one size fits all" approach to determining energy and nutrient needs; the nutrition prescription is highly individualized.

DETERMINING SPECIFIC FEEDING NEEDS

ORAL

FOOD CONSISTENCIES NECESSARY FOR PATIENTS WITH POOR DENTITION

Older adults may experience partial tooth loss or complete tooth loss that requires dentures to help with proper chewing. Individuals with missing teeth and those with dentures or with poorly fitting dentures may have their nutritional intake adversely affected. The intake of fruits, vegetables, and meats may especially be compromised because these foods tend to be more difficult to chew. Often, with poor dentition, a mechanical soft diet is ordered. Foods are typically chopped and/or ground, making chewing less cumbersome. Because nutrition and intake may already be compromised in the elderly, it is especially important for the dietitian to assess chewing ability during the assessment phase.

CLEAR LIQUID DIET AND A FULL LIQUID DIET

A clear liquid diet consists of clear liquids such as fruit juice, tea, and broth. The clear liquid diet may be ordered postsurgery and should only be used short term. The clear liquid diet is severely lacking in adequate energy and nutrients and should only be used on a short-term basis. The patient may be advanced to a full liquid diet if clear liquids are tolerated. Full liquid diets are more substantial and filling than are clear liquid diets. Thicker, heavier liquids such as milk, yogurt, pudding, and creamy soups are typical on a full liquid regimen. Although the full liquid diet provides more calories and nutrients than the clear liquid diet, it is still inadequate and should not be used for more than a few days.

ADHERING TO A DIETARY SCHEDULE

A specific dietary intake schedule or pattern may be useful in a variety of circumstances. After bariatric surgery, patients may benefit from test meals to determine tolerance followed by the initiation of several small meals daily. Individuals who have had bariatric surgery have a smaller stomach "pouch" and are unable to tolerate large amounts of food in one sitting. Diabetic patients are in another group that benefits from a set schedule. For diabetics, consistent carbohydrate intake is essential and helps control hypoglycemia. Patients who have a loss of appetite due to increased age or chronic disease may also benefit from a meal schedule. Several smaller meals daily or meals with snacks can be useful in helping patients achieve adequate nutritional intake.

FOOD SUPPLEMENTS

Oral nutrition supplements can help patients who may otherwise be unable to meet nutrient needs achieve adequate nutrition. Frequently, during the hospital stay the dietitian will recommend oral nutrition supplements such as Boost, Ensure, and high-calorie puddings. Malnutrition is a major concern among elderly patients. Often, upon assessment it is determined the patient is underweight, or inadequate intake may be noted after hospital admission. Preventing and treating malnutrition has a positive impact on outcomes. Elderly patients may suffer from poor dentition, lack of appetite, altered small/taste, and chronic disease, making sufficient intake from meals a challenge. This type of patient generally benefits from food product supplementation. Food supplements may also be used for other patients with malnutrition and poor intake; food supplements may also be added to provide extra nutrients for patients with cancer and those in recovery from surgery, burns, or other wounds.

Benefits of Breastfeeding

Breastfeeding is considered the preferred and best form of nutrition for an infant. Ideally, mothers will breastfeed throughout the first year of life, but it is important to support the mother throughout the process because breastfeeding for shorter periods of time still offers health benefits to the mother and child. Not only is breastmilk designed to meet the nutrient needs of the infant, but breastmilk also offers important immune protection by delivering antibodies from the mother to the infant. Breastfed infants have been shown to have decreased rates of food allergies, asthma, and diabetes. Breastfeeding has benefits for the mother as well, such as helping with postpartum weight loss and reducing rates of hormonal cancers. Beyond the individual benefits, overall healthcare costs can be reduced when breastfeeding occurs.

Breastfeeding Support and Management

The dietitian can support the breastfeeding mother through support and education. Reassuring the mother that breastfeeding is meeting her baby's needs may be necessary. Breastfed infants are typically fed on demand, and unlike feeding with a bottle, the mother does not know how much the baby consumed in a feeding. Breastfeeding infants are expected to have at least five wet diapers daily and three stools per day. These output markers along with monitored weight gain of the infant indicate to the mother that feeding is adequate. Also, it is important to discuss the use of a breast pump with the mother. Breast pumps allow mothers to express milk for later use. This can be helpful when the mother returns to work or needs to be away from the infant for longer than a couple of hours. It is important for the breastfeeding mother to care for herself as well. Breastfeeding is an energy-demanding process, and lactating mothers may require up to 400 additional calories per day.

Enteral and Parenteral Nutrition

Tube Feedings

Several companies manufacture tube feeding products; each facility will choose which formulas that they make available for patients. Standard formulas work best for patients who have a properly functioning digestive system. Elemental formulas are more easily digested and may be appropriate for individuals with compromised digestion such as those with pancreatitis. Specialized formulas are also available, and these formulas are available for patients with a specific medical diagnosis such as diabetes. A person with diabetes might be given a special feeding with fewer carbohydrates. Renal patients on dialysis may benefit from formulas providing increased calories and protein. High-fiber formulas are available and may be chosen for patients experiencing chronic constipation. Also, homemade tube feedings are sometimes used when a patient receives enteral nutrition at home.

Determining the Correct Amounts for Tube Feedings

The amount of tube feeding administered will depend upon the needs of the patient. The dietitian should calculate the energy and nutrient needs in the assessment; an appropriate formula should then be selected. Most enteral formulas are packaged in 240 ml cans. A standard formula provides 1 kcal per milliliter, so a standard formula will contain 240 kcals. Specialized formulas may provide more calories, such as 1.5 or 2.0 kcals per milliliter. Determine the total volume of formula necessary to meet needs. Let us assume that the patient's needs are estimated to be 1,800 kcals/day. For a standard formula, the kcal needs will equal the volume. 1,800 kcals required = 1,800 mL because the standard formula provides 1 kcal per milliliter. If using a specialized formula higher in calories such as 1.5 kcals/mL, the number of kcals needed should be divided by kcals/mL

(1,800 kcals ÷ 1.5 kcals/mL = 1,200 mL total volume per 24-hour period). If the patient will receive a standard formula of four bolus feedings/day, you need to determine the volume administered per feeding. This is calculated as follows:

1,800 mL/day ÷ four feedings per day = 450 mL/feeding.

Situations to Use Parenteral Nutrition

Parenteral nutrition is intravenous nutrition. This type of delivery may be necessary for patients who have altered gut function such as those who have undergone bowel surgery. Parenteral nutrition may be central parenteral nutrition in which placement is in a central vein or peripheral parenteral nutrition in which placement is in a small vein. Central placement allows the patient to receive a higher calorie and osmolarity solution versus peripheral placement. Parenteral nutrition may be infused continuously or in cycles. Commercially available solutions may be used, or pharmacies may compound specific parenteral solutions. Parenteral nutrition requirements should be calculated based on individual patient needs.

Access and Ending Points

Enteral nutrition or tube feedings make use of the gastrointestinal tract. Nasogastric tubes (NGT) are used when feeding needs are short-term. NGTs are placed in the nasal cavity, and the tube ends in the stomach. Similar to NGTs but with different ending points, nasoduodenal tubes and nasojejunal tubes may also be used and are considered short-term feeding modalities. When long-term solutions to feeding are needed, a permanent access point for tube feedings may be surgically placed. The process is known as percutaneous endoscopic gastrostomy (PEG) or percutaneous endoscopic jejunostomy (PEJ). A gastrostomy tube ends in the stomach, and a jejunostomy tube ends in the jejunum.

Administering Tube feedings

Tube feeding frequency depends largely upon what the patient is able to tolerate. Patients who are unable to tolerate large feedings at one time may require continuous feedings using an enteral pump. Intermittent feedings are provided several times per day and may be a better, more flexible option for some patients compared to continuous feeding. Intermittent feedings are administered via drip or pump. Bolus feedings can be used for patients with adequate digestive abilities. Bolus feedings require that the patient tolerate large feedings in a short period of time.

Complications Associated with Enteral and Parenteral Nutrition

Complications from enteral and parenteral nutrition should be monitored. Some typical gastrointestinal problems from enteral feedings include abdominal pain, upset stomach with nausea/vomiting, constipation, and diarrhea. It is important to assess whether these issues are a result of the tube feeding or other factors such as medications or illness. Risk of aspiration is also a concern with enteral nutrition; the patient's bed may be elevated to help reduce this risk. Infections at the site of tube placement may also occur. The dietitian should monitor whether the enteral nutrition is meeting the nutrient needs of the patient. The weight should be measured frequently, actual intake and output should be noted, and the patient should be monitored for overhydration or dehydration. A common and dangerous concern for patients receiving parenteral nutrition is infection. Also, refeeding syndrome can occur in patients who were previously malnourished.

Integrative and Functional Care, Herbal Therapy

Herbal and Dietary Supplements

Integrative medicine is outside of the mainstream and may be used in conjunction with conventional therapies. Examples of integrative therapy include acupuncture, homeopathy, use of botanicals, and chiropractic treatments. The use of integrative therapies is becoming increasingly popular. Dietary supplements may be used to enhance one's nutrition status; the multivitamin is a common supplement used. With so many different kinds and dosages of supplements available over the counter, the public is often not well informed. The Food and Drug Administration and the Federal Trade Commission provide regulation of the dietary supplement industry. Unlike medicines, dietary supplements are not required to undergo rigorous testing prior to being sold to the public. In fact, it must be proven that dietary supplements are unsafe before they may be removed from the market. Dietary supplements that have a long history of safety may be classified as generally recognized as safe (GRAS). Botanical or herbal supplements are derived from plants; examples include echinacea and gingko biloba. In general, the dietitian should urge caution with the use of dietary supplements. The recommendation for supplement use should be based on sound science, and the assessment should include potential drug-nutrient interactions.

Popular Dietary Supplements

Popular dietary supplements and their proposed benefits/uses:

- Calcium: treatment and prevention of osteoporosis
- Iron: prescribed to correct iron-deficiency anemia
- Vitamin D: prescribed when levels are low possibly due to malabsorption
- Fish oil: dyslipidemia and heart disease
- Probiotics: diarrhea treatment and gastrointestinal function
- Chamomile: anxiety
- Ginkgo biloba: improve memory and cognitive function
- Green tea: cardiovascular function
- Garlic: atherosclerosis
- St. John's wort: depression

Implementing Care Plans

Nutrition Therapy for Specific Nutrition-Related Problems

The Nutrition Care Process (NCP) focuses on quality and outcomes through the use of evidence-based practices. Although dietitians have long applied evidence to their practice, a standardized process was lacking. The NCP approach and subsequent standardized documentation links the nutrition diagnosis, intervention, and outcome. When a practitioner uses standardized language to document, it is easier to link interventions to outcomes. Without the use of standardized language and a clear process, proving that the nutrition intervention is an essential service becomes more difficult. Two dietitians may have taken the same action with a patient, yet it may have been documented very differently. With the implementation of standardized language, tracking of nutrition diagnoses and subsequent outcomes become much less complicated and much more reliable. When dietitians use standardized nutrition diagnoses such as "Excessive carbohydrate intake for a type 2 diabetic," the existence of a nutrition problem is clearly pinpointed, and that nutrition diagnosis can be used to track improvements in the patient's status. Although it may not be thought of in these terms, healthcare is a business. The services provided must be cost-effective while bringing about a desired outcome in the patient's health status. Nutrition intervention is effective, and the NCP provides a better means of illustrating the positive impact of the profession.

Counseling and Training

The dietitian is often called upon to train patients so that the education that is provided may be properly implemented. For example, diabetic patients require training in carbohydrate counting and food serving sizes. For individuals discharged on tube feeding, training regarding pump use, administration of feeding, and sanitation will be required. Many patients will benefit from learning how to read food labels and identify serving sizes (for example, a serving size of meat is 3 oz., which is about the size of a deck of cards). Some patients may also benefit from training in healthy cooking techniques and food safety procedures. It is imperative to properly document in the medical record any education and training provided by the dietitian and to whom it was provided (i.e. patient, family members, other caregivers).

Discharge Planning and Disease Management

Referrals for Discharged Patients

The referrals needed may depend on the medical diagnosis, the patient's resources, and physical abilities. For example, a newly diagnosed diabetic will need a referral to an outpatient diabetes education program. Elderly low-income individuals will benefit from a referral to the USDA Commodity Supplemental Food Program to have food delivered to the home. Elderly or disabled patients who are unable to shop for food and cook may require a referral to home service agencies that help with cooking, cleaning, and shopping needs. If depression or another mental health disorder is present, a referral to outpatient psychological services will be warranted. It is important that once the patient leaves the hospital, the continuity of care continues.

MyPlate and Dietary Guidelines for Americans

MyPlate

MyPlate is a guidance system initiated by the United States Department of Agriculture (USDA) in 2011 aimed at encouraging healthy intake. MyPlate replaced MyPyramid, and before that was the Food Guide Pyramid. MyPlate uses a simple plate and cup graphic to encourage variety. As illustrated on the MyPlate graphic, fruits and vegetables should make up half the plate. This illustration emphasizes the importance of fruit and vegetable intake, which is generally lacking in the American diet. The other half of the plate is composed of protein and grains, whereas the cup graphic features dairy. The program encourages intake of lean proteins and whole grains. MyPlate is an easy-to-understand visual that can be used to illustrate how healthy, adequate nutrition intake can be obtained through variety in meals.

Dietary Guidelines for Americans

The Dietary Guidelines for Americans are published every five years by the USDA and the United States Department of Health and Human Services (HHS). The latest edition is the 2015–2020 release. These guidelines are used to develop public policy and establish or improve public programs. The dietary guidelines acknowledge the high incidence of chronic disease related to poor dietary intake. The latest guidelines attempt to provide recommendations in line with addressing this matter. The current guidelines focus on healthy intake and variety, and they encourage a limited intake of added sugars, sodium, and saturated fat.

State and Community Resources and Nutrition-Related Programs

Federal- and State-Funded Food and Nutrition Programs

Women, Infants, and Children Program

The **Women, Infants, and Children (WIC) Program** is funded through a federal grant, and it provides services for low-income pregnant/postpartum women, infants, and children. Services are available during pregnancy, up to a year postpartum if breastfeeding, and for infants and children through five years of age. Not only must participants meet income requirements set by the state, but participants must also be at nutritional risk to be eligible. Examples of nutritional risk include overweight, underweight, or a gestational diabetes diagnosis. If eligible, the participant will receive vouchers to purchase foods. Examples of foods available for purchase include infant formula, baby food, cereals, fruit juice, milk, cheese, peanut butter, fruits, and vegetables. The WIC Program has shown positive intervention outcomes such as a reduced incidence of low-birth weight babies and premature births, improvements in dietary intake, increases in breastfeeding rates, and a reduction in healthcare costs after birth.

Supplemental Nutrition Assistance Program

The **Supplemental Nutrition Assistance Program (SNAP)** is a program administered by the United States Department of Agriculture (USDA) for low-income individuals. Although there are some exclusions, to be eligible for SNAP, those who are able must hold a job. SNAP can be used to buy necessary food for the household, but participants cannot purchase alcoholic beverages or tobacco. There are no restrictions on the type of food that can be purchased, which means that items of little nutritive value such as soft drinks and cakes may be bought. Some farmers' markets accept SNAP benefits, and this is a win-win for consumers and farmers. Consumers get access to high-quality, locally grown fruits and vegetables, and farmers are compensated for their hard work.

Nutrition Programs for Seniors/Older Adults

Block grants are large sums of money allocated to states or territories, and the state or territory has some discretion about how that program-specific grant is to be used. Although the grant must be used for the defined purpose and is subject to specific guidelines, how it is administered is up to the state. Many programs are funded or partially funded through block grants.

The **Senior Farmers' Market Nutrition Program** operates via a federal grant and is administered by individual states. Low-income individuals 60 years of age or older may be eligible. The **Elderly Nutrition Program** is another federal grant program for seniors 60 years of age or older. Although having a low income is not a requirement, the program is marketed toward this group. This program is unique in that it delivers meals to home- or community-based settings such as senior centers. This is especially important because many elderly persons have transportation limitations and mobility issues. The **USDA Commodity Supplemental Food Program** is another service aimed at low-income seniors. This program provides food packages including items such as peanut butter, cereal, canned meats, canned fruits, and canned vegetables.

National School Lunch Program

The National School Lunch Program is a federally funded program under the United States Department of Agriculture (USDA) umbrella. The program provides free or reduced lunch to low-income students in elementary through high school. Schools participating in the program must serve foods that meet federal nutrition requirements. Enrolled schools receive both cash and USDA foods as part of the participation process. The Summer Food Service Program is also a program of the USDA; it provides meals during the summer to low-income students at various participating sites.

Maternal and Child Block Grant

The Maternal and Child Block Grant is provided by the federal government to the states; in turn, the states are also required to provide funds to pay for the programs set forth. The broad objective of the grant is to improve healthcare for low-income women and children. States are given some discretion in how the funds are used; each state may have somewhat different needs to address. Some services offered include newborn screenings, prenatal care, family planning, and oral health, but states can use the funds to create programs and offer services that are priorities for that state.

Medicare and Medicaid

Medicare is government-funded health insurance for seniors. Medicare part A covers hospital stays, and part B covers outpatient services such as a check-up from the primary care physician and medical equipment. Medicare part D covers prescriptions. Medicare part C is a comprehensive plan provided by private insurers who contract with the government to manage the plan.

Medicaid is a health insurance program funded by the federal government and the states. Medicaid provides health insurance primarily for low-income families, pregnant women, children, and medically fragile individuals.

Community Interventions

Homeless individuals would benefit from community nutrition services. Being homeless, these individuals do not have the means to properly prepare meals, and they often go without food. Shelters, food banks, and feeding stations benefit those who do not have access to good-quality food. Low-income individuals also benefit from community nutrition services. Although they may have funds to purchase some foods, often there is not enough money to meet all their needs. Food banks provide a much-needed service to these families who struggle to make ends meet. Certain communities have specific needs, and targeting services to meet those priority needs is desirable. For instance, when conducting a community needs assessment, you may determine that your community has a higher rate of diabetes than the surrounding area. Nutrition services and education aimed at diabetes prevention and treatment would be an appropriate intervention service to offer.

Identification and Attainment of Funding

Once a community intervention need is identified, it may be a challenge to identify and obtain funding sources. Government grants, private grants, and corporate sponsorships all should be considered. Fundraising is another potential source of dollars. After funding sources are secured, a budget should be developed to allocate funds. The budget is a plan or a guide for how resources will be allocated to accomplish objectives and how money will be spent. The budget should point out any potential cash shortfalls that may occur and should indicate if funds will be appropriate to meet needs.

Provision of Food and Nutrition Services to Groups

As with any program, it is important to determine whether objectives are being met and if quality standards are achieved. Once established, it may take time to see a real, widespread impact. Programs hope to address the public health concern for which they were developed. For example, suppose you initiated a community program to curb obesity in a small community. Based on survey data, you knew that the population is low income and has a high rate of obesity. First, in order to make an impact, the message must reach the community. Assume that several members of the community choose to participate in the weight loss program and many more are referred by the local physician. At the first session, everyone is weighed for a baseline measurement. The team of nutrition leaders provides education and tools for healthy eating and physical activity guidance. Weekly, participants check in to get weighed and receive education and encouragement. At the end of three months, the weight loss program concludes, and final weights are measured. At this point, you can determine whether the initial objectives of the program have been met and evaluate how to make improvements for the future.

Monitoring and Evaluation

Monitoring and Evaluating Tolerance to Interventions

Monitoring and Evaluation of the Nutrition Care Process

Monitoring and evaluation is the fourth step in the nutrition care process. In this phase, you compare outcomes to interventions by collecting information that measures progress. It is important to monitor and evaluate the process because you want to know if your intervention is working. If it is not working, changes should be made, and if it is working, this too is vital information because goals are being met. Suppose your patient is obese and a weight loss goal of five pounds within one month was agreed upon. During this phase, you will weigh the patient and compare the current weight with the initial weight. Has the goal been met? If yes, the intervention is working. If the goal is not met, it should be determined whether there was any improvement. For example, suppose the patient lost four pounds but did not reach the goal of losing five pounds. In this case, there was improvement. If the patient lost no weight or gained weight, there was no improvement. It is important to determine why the goal was not met and document these reasons.

Indicators in Evidence-Based Guidelines for Practice

A nutrition indicator is what you will measure. If you are unable to measure, it will be difficult to provide evidence that the intervention is working. Measurable indicators include height, weight, and BMI. Laboratory measurements such as A1C, glucose, and lipids are measurable. Food intake and levels of physical activity are also measurable indicators along with physical appearance and appetite. If the measurable indictor for the patient is the A1C level, it is important to choose the correct standard of reference. A1C goals will differ for diabetic versus nondiabetic patients. Suppose your diabetic patient did not reach his/her set A1C goal for the past three-month period. Any variance from the expected or desired outcome should be explained. Perhaps the patient was on a two-month-long vacation to Europe and did not desire to follow the meal plan. Alternatively, it may be determined that the patient did not have a good understanding of carbohydrate counting and serving sizes, so education and reinforcement will be needed.

Direct Nutrition Outcomes

Nutrition outcomes evaluation will depend upon what is being evaluated. If the patient has excess energy intake and is overweight as evidenced by a BMI of 32, the dietitian can evaluate caloric intake via a food recall or food journal and measure weight to determine BMI. When the diabetic patient has a nutrition diagnosis of excess carbohydrate intake as evidenced by a 24-hour food recall and A1C of 8.2, the outcomes to be measured are carbohydrate intake and A1C. If a post-stroke patient has a nutrition diagnosis of swallowing difficulty, it is important to note that the dietitian cannot correct swallowing problems. The dietitian can recommend the appropriate dysphagia diet and monitor/evaluate tolerance. Although the swallowing difficulty may persist or resolve, the dietitian must address the signs or symptoms of dysphagia, such as food avoidance or choking/coughing while eating. The dietitian should prescribe a diet that minimizes swallowing difficulty and is nutritionally adequate, so those are the outcomes that would be evaluated.

Clinical/Health Status Outcomes and Patient-Centered Outcomes

Patient-centered care focuses on factors that are important to the patient as opposed to simply focusing on factors relevant to the provider of services. If an intervention or treatment is important to the patient, conceivably this may help bring about a better outcome. Let us assume that our patient is obese and has also recently been diagnosed with type 2 diabetes. The patient admits to struggling with weight for years, but recently he has become very unhappy with his increased weight and wants to reach a healthier weight. He wants to look and feel better. In this scenario, weight loss is important to the patient, so he may be more likely to take steps needed for weight loss. Improving diet and increasing physical activity to promote weight loss will likely also lead to improvements in blood glucose control (a clinical outcome). In this scenario, addressing a patient-centered outcome offers many potential benefits. Although there has generally been a focus on clinical outcomes (laboratory tests, symptom improvement, etc.), when possible, a patient-centered focus should be incorporated into care.

Healthcare Utilization Outcomes

Healthcare utilization is the use of healthcare services. It is important that the services offered, rendered, and paid for provide positive, cost-effective solutions to problems. Payors such as Medicare, Medicaid, and private insurers are concerned with the effectiveness and cost of services. If services are to be paid for, they are expected to provide value by having a positive impact on the health problem. For instance, if nutrition services are to be covered for a type 2 diabetic, one would expect to see an improvement in blood glucose levels leading to better management of symptoms. This is important because the patient wants to see improvement in his or her health and quality of life. It is also important because payors responsible for reimbursement must justify payment because healthcare costs must be controlled. So, if nutrition services help the diabetic patient as evidenced by better blood sugar control, a number of factors become important. Better blood glucose control can reduce the need for prescription medications, and it can reduce the risk of diabetic complications such as neuropathy, retinopathy, and cardiovascular disease. Clearly, these outcomes are positive for the patient and are cost-effective.

Outcome Measurement and Quality Improvement

By measuring outcomes, you can determine if the intervention is working, and if the intervention is not working, you can make a plan to correct it. Unless you evaluate outcomes, you don't really know if the intervention is successful. For example, suppose you recommend a 2,000-calorie diabetic diet to a newly diagnosed, overweight type 2 diabetic. In theory, if the patient follows the 2,000-calorie meal plan that is prescribed, the blood glucose levels should improve. There are many reasons why blood glucose levels may not improve with the prescribed diet, and you cannot know the result unless it is measured. In three months, when you follow up with your diabetic patient, you determine that the postprandial blood glucose levels are too high, weight loss has not occurred, and A1C has not improved. Upon reassessment, you determine that the patient needed further diabetes diet education and a reduction in calories. The meal plan was changed to an 1,800-calorie diabetic diet. At the following six-month follow-up visit, the patient had lost 12 pounds and had vastly improved blood glucose and A1C levels. Measuring outcomes provides an opportunity to make changes and adjustments to care plans, thus improving the quality of the healthcare that is provided.

Determining Whether Care Should Be Continued, Changed, or Discontinued

When comparing outcomes with interventions during the monitoring and evaluation phase, you have an opportunity to update the care plan as needed. When evaluating, it may be determined that improvement is being made and care should continue. Likewise, the dietitian may also note that there is no improvement or improvement is not as expected and goals are not met. In this case, it is necessary to reassess the patient to determine why goals are not being met. Perhaps there is a lack of understanding with the patient, or the nutrition prescription may need altering to better meet needs in order to achieve the goal. Finally, if the goals have been met and the issues are resolved, care can be discontinued.

Management of Food and Nutrition Programs and Services

Functions of Management

Planning

Short- and Long-Term

Short-term planning, as the name implies, is planning for a time period in the near future. Short-term plans look at the coming year. A short-term goal might be to hire extra staff for the busy season.

Long-term planning looks further into the future than short-term planning. It tends to have a broader focus and looks at organizational goals and needs. When planning for the long term and looking ahead several years, you must anticipate future needs. If you need additional space to serve your clients or customers, a long-term plan could be to relocate, expand, or build a new facility.

Strategic and Operational

A **strategic plan** is a long-term plan that involves analyzing your current position and looks into the future to where you envision the organization. The strategic plan has a goal-setting and goal-achieving focus for the future. If healthcare is your business, you will want to observe industry trends and visualize the future of healthcare. Strategic planning involves how you will achieve your long-term goals. The same is true for foodservice management: managers must try to plan for future changes and align the organization in a way to meet those future goals and to stay competitive. **Operational planning** involves more short-term, day-to-day activities and may be department specific rather than having a company-wide focus. Operational plans should help organizations reach their strategic goals.

Policies and Procedures

A **policy** could be described as what should be done, and a **procedure** is how something is done. Policies and procedures are in place to maintain quality, consistency, and safety in the work environment. Policies and procedures can help prevent chaos, costly mistakes, and disorganization by communicating organization expectations to employees. Upon hire, most employees are required to read the employee handbook, which outlines the policies of the organization. Policies may include proper work attire, attendance requirements, and workplace behavior. Policies and procedures in a healthcare environment are necessary to protect employees and patients. For example, in a hospital there are specific procedures that healthcare professional must follow to do their jobs safely and effectively. The same is true in a foodservice organization. Employees must follow certain procedures to safely prepare and serve meals.

Emergency Preparedness

Emergencies may take many forms. Natural disasters occur in the form of floods and tornados, whereas other emergencies may come in the form of terrorism or an intruder. Organizations must have plans in place to address potential emergencies for the safety of their employees, patients, and the public at large. A cornerstone of emergency management is to be prepared in case disaster strikes. Although preventing an emergency situation is not always possible, part of the plan focuses on prevention. Obviously, in the case of a natural disaster, prevention is not possible, but it may be possible to suppress an intruder and limit casualties or property damage. Part of being prepared is knowing how to behave when emergencies arise. This preparedness can include active shooter training, fire drills, or bomb drills. Individuals need to know what to do and where to go in the case of an emergency. Finally, there needs to be a plan for how to recover once the emergency is over. For instance, if massive flooding requires the operation to shut down, there should be procedures in place detailing how and when operations will resume.

Organizing

Schedules and Full-Time Equivalent (FTE) Allocations

Having employees present at work when they are needed is essential in all businesses. This requires planning employee schedules and anticipating work needs. Organizing schedules might be rather easy when needs vary little and the typical workday is 8:00 a.m. to 5:00 p.m. In the case of foodservice organizations, needs may be more variable. Individuals may need to be scheduled for the breakfast shift, lunch run, or dinner. Depending on the menu and number of patrons, prep and cook times will vary and schedules must be adjusted accordingly.

Some employers, such as foodservice operations, may employ several part-time employees. A manager may need to know how these part-time employees compare with having full-time employees. A full-time employee typically works 40 hours a week or 2,080 hours per year. You can calculate full-time equivalents (FTEs) for your employees. If you wish to calculate annual FTEs and know the total number of labor hours, divide that number by 2,080. For example, assume that all of your employees worked a total of 30,000 hours in a year: 30,000 ÷ 2,080 = 14.42 FTEs.

Department or Unit Structure

Organizations, departments, or unit structures may be illustrated using an **organizational chart**. The organizational chart shows where an employee fits within the department or within the organization. The chart generally details individuals in management at the top of the chart and shows the employee function/title that falls under each manager. The organizational chart shows a snapshot of the organization and illustrates reporting functions. **Line** positions are those functions that relate directly to the customer; this might be a worker on the serving line. **Staff** functions do not have a direct impact on the customer; these roles may be found in departments such as finance or accounting.

Organizations can be structured as **centralized** or **decentralized**. In centralized organizations, most decisions are made by top management, but in decentralized organizations, decision are spread among lower level managers and departments. A decentralized organization gives departments or units greater control over their areas.

Processes, Procedures, and Improving Productivity

Organizations are expected to produce, whether it is a physical good or a service. A function of management is to facilitate production. One such way to develop processes and procedures for how things are done is to set goals. One way to help achieve goals is through training and education. A lack of training can hinder productivity and overall efficiency. Another key to productively is effective communication. In order to achieve productivity goals, employees need to understand the expectations and requirements of their jobs. This includes overall expectations and, in some cases, daily tasks. In addition, the manager should make sure that working conditions and equipment are up to date for optimized productivity.

Resources

Resources that need to be managed include time, money, people, and technology. Effective resource management can affect productivity. Technology is a resource that can be used to effectively facilitate and streamline jobs. When managed appropriately and with proper employee training, technology can be an asset to an organization. Time is a resource because it is not unlimited, and most workplaces expect a certain amount of productivity within a given period of time. Financial resources are also important because most departments have a finite budget; how those funds are used can ultimately impact productivity. Using money wisely to invest in other resources is a management function. Finally, people and their skills are resources that must be managed in order to reach department and organization objectives.

DIRECTING

COORDINATION AND DELEGATION

Coordination of people and groups along with delegation are functions of management. People or groups need to be coordinated in order to achieve a specific objective. If the objective is preparing and delivering the dinner meal for patients, resources must be coordinated to prep, cook, plate, and deliver. Managers must also be good delegators of authority and tasks; it takes multiple people to accomplish most major objectives. When you delegate, you entrust in others and empower them. Through delegation, employees learn responsibility and new skills. When a manager delegates, he/she must communicate the expectations and provide the necessary direction for the employee to complete the task.

COMMUNICATION

COMMUNICATION BARRIERS

Communication is more than just saying words; it is an effective exchange of information. Sometimes, we receive too much information and it is difficult to distinguish what is truly important. At other times, not enough information is conveyed, and this can leave one in a state of confusion or unknowing. Individuals may also "hear what they want to hear." We may put our own spin on words even though that was not the intended meaning. At other times, we simply fail to listen, and the message is not received. Furthermore, individuals have different communication styles, and people respond in various ways. Effective communication can be challenging, and it is important to recognize and try to overcome these barriers.

TYPES OF COMMUNICATION

Communication can be verbal, nonverbal, or written — but all of these forms provide information to the receiver. Verbal communication uses words to exchange information. This could be a face-to-face exchange, via telephone, or videoconference. Nonverbal communication does not use words; rather, it uses gestures and body language. Your posture and facial expressions can communicate a lot about how you are feeling. Written communication takes many forms and has many purposes. Company policies and procedures are generally written and are often available via paper forms or an employee intranet. Email and texting provide an avenue for written communications. These avenues can increase efficiency for organizations when used appropriately.

MOTIVATIONAL STRATEGIES

Maslow's hierarchy of needs: This theory by Abraham Maslow says that basic needs must be met before a person will focus on higher level needs. Physiological needs are the basis of the hierarchy; physiological needs such as food may be linked to survival. If someone is starving, he/she is likely to focus on this need rather than higher order needs such as self-esteem. Once a lower level need is met, the focus can shift to higher level needs.

Two-factor theory: This theory by Frederick Herzberg looks at things that satisfy and things that dissatisfy. Hygiene factors, such as salary and working environment, can cause dissatisfaction in the workplace. Interestingly, the absence of these factors does not result in satisfaction — you expect a reasonable salary and good working conditions. Motivating factors such as recognition and growth potential tend to be closely tied to job satisfaction.

Acquired needs theory: Douglas McClelland proposed this theory, which states that people have a need for achievement, power, and affiliation. People who need achievement are very goal oriented. Those who have affiliation needs are concerned about what others think, and those needing power may wish to control situations.

Reinforcement theory: This theory is based on work by B.F. Skinner and Ivan Pavlov; it states that our actions are dictated by what happens as a result of those actions. For example, if we are consistently late to work and there are no consequences, we may continue this trend. Alternatively, if we are late and are reprimanded, this may deter such action.

Leadership Theories

The **great man theory** (proposed in the 1800s) says that some people are born to be leaders rather than developing leadership characteristics throughout life. This theory focuses on natural traits with which many people may be born.

The **trait theory** says that people are born with leadership traits that well prepare them for leadership roles.

Participative leadership theories state that leadership is best when the input of others is sought and put into action.

Situational leadership theories indicate that leadership is dictated by the specific situation. Certain circumstances call for one type of leadership, whereas other circumstances may benefit from a completely different style. In this scenario, leaders adapt their approach and style. This is similar to **contingency theory**, which also focuses on circumstances/events rather than one leadership style or approach.

Transformation leadership can truly transform an organization or department. Transformational leaders can inspire and motivate employees.

Management Theories

Theory of scientific management by Frederick Taylor focuses on four aspects of work. First, the focus is on finding novel ways to do the job. Sometimes processes can be improved with a new approach. Second, train the employee. Third, the employer and employee should have similar goals. Finally, reward high performers with monetary compensation.

Administrative management theory by Henri Fayol developed principles and functions of management. Principles include authority and initiative, whereas functions include planning and organizing. Fayol's contributions have helped shaped how management is viewed today.

Bureaucratic theory of management by Max Weber looked at the difference between power and authority. This approach takes a strict view of management and focuses on rules and tasks to create optimal work output.

Management by objectives by Peter Drucker focuses on alignment of employee and organization goals to achieve objectives.

Controlling

Establishing Standards, Monitoring Established Plans, and Developing Corrective Actions

Controlling is a function of management that includes establishing standards, performance evaluation, and corrective action if needed. Each business may have different standards by which employees abide. In foodservice and healthcare, there will be quality and safety standards that must be met. In addition, in many organizations, there are financial and productivity standards. Performance evaluations will include how well the employee adheres to the standards. Employees might be evaluated on productivity based on sales figures. Other employees might be evaluated on the basis of adhering to safety protocols. If there are deviations from the standard or goals are not met, corrective action may need to be taken.

Staffing

Forecasting Personnel Needs and Alignment of Personnel

It is important to anticipate the number of employees you need for any given day or task so that production needs can be met. Hiring too many employees could mean that there is not enough work for everyone, and having too few staff members working can put a stress on existing personnel and production may not be met. Historical data may help with forecasting staffing needs. If in the past you have needed four full-time dietitians when the census is average, this information can help predict future needs. Of course, you must also consider scenarios in which the census is above average and take into account work absences. In addition, staffing needs may also change when the organization expands. Perhaps the hospital is building a new week to accommodate more beds; you will likely need to expand your staff based on anticipated future needs. Managers must also align personnel to meet the goals of the organization and department. Skills and abilities should be aligned with the job tasks for optimal performance and outcome.

Skills

Technical

The technical skills required for a job may vary depending on the managerial role. Some roles will require more technical expertise than others, but having technical skills is an asset for managers. Not only can these skills be useful in your specific management functions, but it can also be helpful to have the technical know-how to understand your employees' functions.

Technical skills may include an understanding of how equipment works in the foodservice operation. Other technical skills include familiarity with technology such as computers and tablets. Many forms of communication rely on technology, and the manager should have adequate skills to use technology appropriately. In general, higher level managers may not need the technical expertise that may benefit lower level managers.

Human and Conceptual

Typically, to be truly effective, managers must interact with and manage people. Therefore, having interpersonal skills is essential. As a manager, you need to be able to relate to your employees, and this may help them relate to you. People are much different than technology; we can program devices to behave in a certain manner, but humans are more complex. Managers must employ human skills to direct, lead, and motivate individuals in order to accomplish goals. There are many different interpersonal skills that can be beneficial for managers. Managers should have the ability to communicate effectively and respectfully. Managers should be understanding and possess the ability to listen. Finally, managers should have the ability to bring together teams to accomplish a common goal. Conceptual skills include seeing the big picture — this goes well beyond the day-today activities. A conceptual skill includes a manager's ability to understand how their unit's role fits into the goals of the organization. Conceptual skills can be useful in strategic planning and goal alignment.

Roles

Informational

Managers wear many hats, and one role is to provide information to employees. Often, organizations have a hierarchy, and information may flow down from one level to another. Policy changes or other pertinent information coming from the top will need to be communicated by the manger to his/her employees. Also, the manager may need to provide department-specific information. If there is a change in processes or updates, the manager provides that information to the employees. Information sharing may also be directed at an individual employee to help him or her become more effective at the job.

Conflict Resolution

Managers must work to resolve conflicts that come up within the organization or specific department. Conflicts come about for many reasons. There may be individual conflicts between employees, or there may be conflicts about goal alignment and the direction that the organization is taking. When conflicts between individual employees arise, managers must seek to resolve them and restore harmony. He or she must be a good listener and take into account all sides of the issue. The conflict may be a misunderstanding or a difference of opinion or way of doing things, or it may involve legal matters. The manager must handle each situation differently and appropriately according to the organization's policies and the law. When conflicts about the direction of the organization arise, an open dialogue is important to allow all voices to be heard.

Problem Solving

Managers are also problem solvers. Frequently, organizations and departments encounter problems or obstacles that make achieving goals difficult. The ability to think creatively and outside the box can help solve problems. If an employee goes to his or her manager and explains that the staff is unable to complete the lunch tasks prior to starting dinner prep, the manager must figure out where the problem lies and determine how to fix it. The answer may be obvious in that lunch prep should begin earlier. The problem may also be broader in nature and require a strategic focus. Perhaps the current foodservice technology system is not meeting the goals of the department. The manager must begin to determine the limitations of the current system and consider whether upgrades or a new system are feasible given the budget.

Decision Making

Managers need to be effective decision makers. The decisions made by mangers can affect the department and the organization as a whole. Management decisions affect employees, customers, patients, and coworkers. Managers are called upon to consider all of the available options and make decisions that benefit the organization.

Traits

Management Styles

Management style and leadership style terminology are often used interchangeably. The following four styles are based on the situational leadership model developed by Paul Hersey.

Coaching offers support and direction; this style works well when the employees are motivated. The manager proactively works as a mentor to help employees achieve their goals.

Directive offers direction but little support; this style works best when employees need a lot of direction or instruction.

Supportive offers little direction but much support; this style may work best when the employees are fairly well trained or experienced.

Delegating offers little direction and little support; this style works well when little supervision is required.

Leadership Styles

Management style and leadership style terminology are often used interchangeably.

Democratic leaders encourage others to participate in the decision-making process. They hear feedback and consider opinions other than their own. This style of leadership exhibits a team approach and makes participants feel valued.

Autocratic leaders do not seek outside opinion or input for decisions. This type of leadership can be suppressive.

Laissez-faire leadership is a very laid back, casual approach to leadership. This leader generally provides little oversight or feedback to employees.

Interpersonal Traits

Although there are numerous personality traits that a person can possess, Lewis Goldberg identified five traits that may be prominent. They are openness, conscientiousness, extraversion, agreeableness, and neuroticism. Individuals who are open may be willing to deviate from the norm and explore better ways of doing things. A conscientious person pays attention to detail and may be structured. Someone who is extraverted tends to be more social and expressive. An agreeable individual generally goes with the flow and tends to be understanding. The neurotic trait may be exhibited in someone who is disruptive and lacking a positive outlook.

Managing a Diverse Workforce

Diversity comes in many forms including gender, race, ethnic, and religion. In the workplace, we are likely to encounter diversity as a coworker and as a manager. Managing diversity can start with understanding diversity. Become educated about what makes people unique. Diversity can bring different perspectives because of different backgrounds, attitudes, or beliefs. Although diversity can bring misunderstandings or conflict in the workplace, an open dialogue can help mitigate those instances. As a manager, try to learn as much as possible about the individuals that you manage, so you can better understand and relate to your team. As always, employees should be treated with respect.

Scope of Practice and Standards of Professional Performance

Professionals should operate within their scope of practice. There are many areas in which dietitians are qualified to practice, and there are some areas that would be considered outside the scope of practice. The Academy of Nutrition and Dietetics addresses the scope of practice and standards of performance for the profession. The academy offers decision tools to help dietitians operate within their scope of practice. According to the academy, the scope of practice, "encompasses the range of roles, activities, and regulations within which nutrition and dietetics practitioners perform." The scope of practice takes into account many considerations including education, credentialing, and competence.

Human Resources

Regulatory Compliance

The **Americans with Disabilities Act (ADA)** seeks to provide equal treatment for individuals affected by a disability. The act prohibits workplace discrimination and public service discrimination for those having a disability. Employers must provide "reasonable accommodations" to employees with a disability to assist them in the workplace. The ADA also dictates accessibility for handicapped persons; this may include parking spaces, ramps, etc.

The **Equal Employment Opportunity Commission** enforces antidiscrimination laws in hiring or employment. Individuals cannot be discriminated against for race, color, religion, sex, age, national origin, or disability. In general, entities that employ greater than 15 people must comply with these regulations.

The **Fair Labor Standards Act** dictates wage and overtime pay standards for nonexempt individuals. It also establishes minimum age work requirements.

The **Uniformed Services Employment and Reemployment Act** says individuals entering the military or those recalled for active duty may legally return to their previous employer after service.

Occupational Safety and Health Act establishes health and safety standards in the workplace.

Unions and Contracts

Labor unions are organized to achieve objectives for employees such as fair working conditions and pay. Unions serve to represent the interest of the employees, but unions and employers often have different views. Most organizations do not have unions, but for those that do, the unions and management must reach a consensus when disagreements arise. The two parties form a contract that details the agreed-upon conditions. These conditions could include a number of items such as paid time off, health insurance, and wages. Management and unions will typically negotiate, which is called collective bargaining, until a formal agreement is reached.

Job Analysis, Job Specifications, and Job Descriptions

A **job analysis** analyzes the functions of a job. It also looks at the work environment, management links, and education/training needed to fulfill the job duties. A job analysis can help make sure that candidates and employees are meeting the needs of the organization and that the organization is meeting the needs of the candidate. Referencing an up-to-date job analysis can be useful when hiring, training, and compensating employees. A job analysis can also help develop **job specifications**. Job specifications are the specifics (skills, education, etc.) of what is needed to fulfill the job duties. Job descriptions are also used to detail many aspects of the job. **Job descriptions** help the employee understand the requirements and expectations of the position. Job descriptions generally detail to whom the employee reports and outlines the functions of the job.

Recruitment and Selection

Employee Recruitment Process

Whether an employee leaves your organization or you are expanding staff, employees will need to be recruited and selected for the job(s). Once you have identified the needs and developed a job description, you can begin the recruitment process. A fundamental question is: How will you reach your intended audience to advertise the job opening? There are many different sources for posting jobs. You may do an internal job post giving organizational employees the first option to be considered for the position. Frequently, you will need to go outside the organization to recruit. Your organization may have a website featuring a career page where employees can directly apply for jobs. Jobs can also be posted on a multitude of recruitment websites. You may also wish to notify your professional organization of the job opening, and in turn they can communicate this opportunity to their membership. Although not as widely used today, newspapers are still a source of job listings. You may also wish to participate in recruitment fairs and use social media to promote your recruitment objectives.

Employee Selection Process

Hopefully, you will have several qualified candidates apply for the position that you posted. At this point, you must begin the careful review of applicants and narrow down the candidates. You will likely wish to contact the candidates and ask for a formal interview. Sometimes, a phone interview is conducted prior to a face-to-face interview. This can be especially helpful if the potential recruit is from out of the area. You should consider who from the organization will attend the interview and how the questions will be structured. You should ask all the candidates the same questions so you can easily compare. Furthermore, avoid questions of a personal nature. Many questions are illegal because it can be discriminatory (even if that is not the intent). For example, you cannot ask about a person's age or their parental status. Once you have identified the final candidates, you may wish to have a second interview if a clear front-runner is not obvious. Finally, before extending an offer of employment, a background check may be necessary, and recruits would need to submit to this requirement.

Orientation and Training

Upon hire, new employees will likely participate in an employee orientation. Although the setup will differ among organizations, the goal is to orient the new employee to the organization and to the specific job. Orientations often include required paperwork, benefits review, and an overview of policies and procedures. Beyond the necessities and legalities, the orientation may also provide the employee with a greater appreciation of the organization by discussing organization's background/history, mission, and core values. New employees will likely meet other employees and learn about various departments within the company. They may also have the opportunity to train with a seasoned employee; this helps the new employees "learn the ropes." Beyond the initial orientation, additional employee training may be provided during employment. Examples of training include diversity training, computer training, and cardiopulmonary resuscitation classes.

Performance Improvement and Development

Often, individuals and organizations want to go beyond the status quo. Organizations can help individuals improve performance and develop skills; this helps the employee and the organization achieve goals. Together, the employee and manager develop a plan to address personal and organizational goals that can be addressed during the process. What are the areas of needed growth? What are the areas in which the employee is excelling? Are there areas in which the employee is performing unsatisfactorily or below expectations? Assessing all of these criteria can help you and the employee write an employee development plan. Perhaps the plan will include additional training or higher education. The goal might be to work on time management or people skills. Once the plan is devised, a follow-up time should be scheduled to discuss progress with the employee.

Discipline

As a manager, it is likely that at some point you will face the need to discipline an employee. The incident may be minor, or it may be a major infraction, but the goal is to deter the behavior and improve the circumstance/situation. For managers, it is important to discipline fairly and quickly. If several employees are consistently taking 20 minutes for their 10-minute break and you only discipline one individual, this is not equitable discipline. At first, you may want to simply speak with the offender and explain the rules and implications. A 10-minute break is allowed and going beyond 10 minutes requires his/her coworkers to fill in and pick up the slack during his/her absence. If the verbal warning does not eliminate the behavior, some organizations will then issue a written warning. A written warning is more formal and may outline consequences if improvement is not noted. Finally, a last warning or probation may be necessary — this provides a final opportunity for change. When a manager has legally followed the discipline process set up by the organization, and the employee fails to alter the behavior, termination may result.

Grievance

In addition to managing day-to-day activities, managers must also deal with employee grievances or complaints. Grievances may be minor, such as the coffee machine is not working, or they may be more serious in nature. Organizations should have grievance policies and procedures in place so when true grievances arise, they may be dealt with appropriately. These policies and procedures should be effectively communicated to employees. Whereas a broken coffee machine may not require a written grievance form, other issues such as employee misconduct or theft will need to be formally documented. Managers should seek to gather the facts and consider any legal issues that may pertain to the grievance. If warranted, higher level managers may also need to be involved in the resolution.

Compensation, Retention, and Turnover

Employees expect to be compensated, or paid, for the work they do. Compensation may also include benefits such as life and health insurance, wellness programs, 401(k)/retirement, and financial bonuses. Inadequate compensation can lead to employee dissatisfaction. In turn, this may lead employees to seek other employment. Organizations are better off when they retain good employees because most likely they have invested in the employee. When an employee leaves the organization, a replacement must be found. It may take time to find a replacement, and in the meantime, you will be understaffed. The new employee will need to be trained and oriented to the organization. Employee turnover can have negative effects on the organization, and it is vital that organizations try to retain employees when possible. The employee turnover rate is calculated as follows:

(Number of employees who left or were terminated ÷ total number of employees in the department) × 100.

For example, if you have 35 employees and 9 employees leave, the turnover rate is $(9 \div 35) \times 100 = 25.7\%$.

Personnel Records

Organizations will have varying requirements for the personnel file, but, in general, the file contains information about the employee. These files should be kept confidential and secured. The human resources department generally maintains personnel files. The files will likely include legal documents completed upon hire, application/resume, information about compensation, job descriptions, promotions, disciplinary action, praises, etc. This file serves as a working reference for the organization. The personnel files may also include a separate medical file and will include an I-9 file, as required by law. An I-9 form is completed by employees to show that he/she may legally work in the United States. These forms are kept separate from other personnel files and may be subject to government inspection.

Financial Management

Budget Procedures

A budget is really a plan, a financial plan for the future. Budgets are used in organizations and individual departments to estimate income and to allocate resources appropriately. Budgeting helps managers understand how the money available can be used to achieve objectives throughout a given budgetary period; it is an important decision-making tool. Without a budget to follow, all resources could be squandered on a particular project while leaving shortfalls for other necessary areas. Budgeting requires individuals in the organization to gather information. You must anticipate how much money will be coming into the organization and how much will be going out. You need to project revenue as well as expenses such as employee payroll. Organizations often use historical data to help anticipate future needs, but there are likely to be changes from one year to the next. You may have additional staffing requirements, or maybe the grant the money you were receiving will not be renewed for the coming year. Some organizations use a budget director and a budget committee to help coordinate the budget process.

Types

Operational

An operating budget is concerned with various areas of the operation, and the focus is on money coming into the organization. An operating budget includes areas of the organization that generate income. Depending on the organization, this may be only one area of the company or multiple areas. Keep in mind, even nonprofit organizations need to generate income to function, and they, too, will have a budget. In a hospital system, many units or departments will generate income. For example, you might expect the foodservice operation and surgery center to generate income (among many others). To budget, you need to anticipate how much money will be brought in for the coming year. You can use historical data as one point of reference, but it is wise to also anticipate changes. Perhaps there is a new hospital in town, and the competition may impact income. Likewise, you have expanded the foodservice operations and now offer a more appealing setup - you anticipate that these new offerings will generate additional income. The operating budget contains many components including sales, material purchases, direct labor, marketing expense, and administrative expenses.

Capital

Capital budgeting looks at large expenses that are anticipated for the coming year or years. These are generally considered long-term investments. Capital expenses include major expenses such as buildings, land, and equipment. For a hospital system, capital investments would be a new wing of the hospital or the purchase of new diagnostic machinery. For the foodservice operation, capital expenses might be the addition of a new built-in freezer or other foodservice equipment. These additions are quite costly, and an organization has to budget for such expenses.

Methods

Incremental

An **incremental budget** draws from the previous year's budget; a large deviation from the last year's income is not expected. This is a fairly quick way to budget when there is little fluctuation from year to year. Your budget for the previous year is likely to look very similar to your budget for the coming year. This type of budget may inadvertently encourage managers to spend the majority of their allotted funds in order to avoid a budget reduction the following year.

PERFORMANCE

The **performance budget** is a different approach to budgeting that attempts to tie expenditures to results (or performance). The idea is to illustrate how spending will produce desired results that are measurable.

ZERO-BASED

Zero-based budgeting is an in-depth approach to budgeting that requires analysis and justification for anticipated expenses.

FLEXIBLE

Flexible budgets provide flexibility in the budget and reflect various activity levels rather than one activity level, as seen in static budgets. If the hospital requires more labor hours during the winter months due to an unusually high census, the flexible budget could reflect this change in activity.

FIXED

A **fixed budget**, also called a static budget, does not change based on the level of activity.

COMPONENTS

TYPES OF EXPENSES

There are many different types of expenses encountered by businesses. Taxes are one type of expense that must always be paid. In addition, organizations must pay utilities and payroll, and they must purchase supplies — these are known as operating expenses. Capital expenses are often incurred when new equipment is purchased, or a major improvement is implemented. Cost of goods sold expenses involve the purchase of materials and the direct labor involved in producing a product. **Fixed costs** are costs that do not vary depending on volume. So, if your foodservice operation only makes 200 meals during the month of July versus the typical 350 meals, you are still required to pay expenses such as insurance and building rent. **Variable costs** do vary depending on the level of activity. If you only serve 200 meals instead of 350, your food costs should decrease (if you are planning well); this is an example of a variable cost.

REVENUE STREAMS AND PROFITABILITY

Revenue streams provide the source(s) of income for a business. Generally, a revenue stream provides continuous income. For instance, a revenue stream for a hospital might be sales from foodservice operations. If you are managing the foodservice operation, you might further define the specifics of your revenue stream to know where you are making the most money (or losing money). Businesses need to have revenue in order to be profitable. Revenue is essentially the sales or money coming into the business. Profit is the money left over after you subtract expenses. Unfortunately, you can have significant revenue along with major expenses and not be profitable; in this case, you are operating at a loss. When you operate at a loss, you spend more money than you take in. As a business, you must be concerned with revenue and expenses to make a profit.

RESOURCE ALLOCATION

As a manager, you should allocate your resources wisely. Investing funds in areas that will further the organization and hopefully maximize productivity and quality will ideally result in maximum income. At the same time, avoid investing in areas with limited growth potential and areas that do not have the desired output. Your budget is a financial plan, and your financial plan should help meet your department's and organization's objectives. Your budget is the document showing the estimated funds available, and it details how resources are allocated.

Cash Control and Auditing

Organizations should have cash control procedures in place to minimize losses. Only certain designated individuals should be allowed access to cash. Those individuals who are granted access should have had a background check and an employment verification history to confirm no prior history of problems. Any discrepancies in cash must be investigated; if your cash on hand does not match your receipts, you must determine why. This may simply be a counting error, but theft can also be a possibility.

Financial Statements and Financial Analysis

Accounting is used by businesses and organizations to keep track of finances and to communicate financial data. Generally accepted accounting principles dictate how financial statements are put together.

The **income statement** shows sales or revenues, expenses, taxes, and a profit or loss (known as net income or loss). The **balance sheet** is useful for entities outside the business in making investment decisions. The balance sheet details the company's assets, liabilities, and owner's equity. The **statement of cash flows** illustrates cash coming into and going out of the business. The **statement of retained earnings** indicates how retained earnings (profits, dividends paid) have changed within a given time period.

Outside investors and internal management will generally use financial statements to analyze the health of a business. Outside investors are interested in whether they should put their assets (money) into a business; before doing so, investors want to make sure the business is financially sound. Management performs analyses to determine how to invest current assets to decide if their investment (perhaps an equipment purchase or a new building) will provide an adequate future return.

Accounting Principles

Accounts receivable (A/R) turnover shows how quickly one collects from credit sales.

A/R turnover = annual credit sales ÷ average accounts payable.

Inventory turnover rate = cost of goods sold ÷ average inventory.

Breakeven (in units) = fixed costs ÷ (sales price – variable costs).

Breakeven (in dollars) = breakeven in units × sales price per unit.

Profit margin = net income ÷ net sales.

Cost-Benefit Analysis

Prior to investing money in a project, equipment, etc., a **cost-benefit analysis** might be conducted to determine if the benefits outweigh the costs. When investing money, you want to see a return on your investment and you expect that the investment will further your business goals. A cost-benefit analysis can help in making this determination. As part of the cost-benefit analysis, you should look at the **opportunity cost**. Opportunity costs are the benefits given up should you proceed with the project in question; in other words, you must consider other ways in which the money can be invested besides the proposed project. Is pursuing the current, proposed project worth the opportunity cost (is it worth what you give up)? Of course, you also want to look at the money the proposed project will bring into the organization. If you are considering a cafeteria expansion, you must consider whether this expansion will produce additional revenue. Also, when will you recoup the investment? The expanded cafeteria will hopefully encourage patrons to visit rather than finding an alternative eatery. Beyond revenue, there are other benefits that may be less obvious. Perhaps the expansion will relieve cafeteria overcrowding and make the employees and visitors happier. In general, when the benefits outweigh the costs, the project may be suitable for the organization.

Marketing and Public Relations

PROCESS

IDENTIFICATION OF TARGET MARKET AND DETERMINATION OF NEEDS/WANTS

A **target market** is a specific group or groups of people to which you wish to market your products or services. These groups generally have specific characteristics that you have identified that would make them potential purchasers of your goods or services. Perhaps your target market has wants or needs for your products or services. Customer wants and needs are very different but wants and needs should be determined during market research. For instance, a consumer may need a healthcare provider, but he or she may want a spa day.

Target marketing is more focused than mass marketing; with target marketing, you focus on a specific group rather than marketing to everyone. In order to market to your target, you must first identify your target market. Who are you trying to reach with your message? This step involves conducting market research. This might include demographics, surveys, and observation. Once you have an idea of who your customer is, you can focus on how to effectively reach that market with your message.

MARKETING MIX

Product, **placement**, **promotion**, and **price** are commonly known as the 4 Ps of marketing. A good marketing mix must encompass these four areas. The product is what you are selling — it may be a physical good or a service you are offering. Hopefully, your product or service will meet a want or a need of your target market. The placement of your goods and services is also important. How will the customer purchase your product or access your service? Is this location convenient, and will it attract your target market? Of course, you will want to promote your product or service. If you are running a restaurant, you want people to know where it is and how to get there. The same is true for a service: You must promote the services you offer and let people know why they want/need what you are offering. There are many ways to promote, including websites, social media, billboards, and word of mouth. Finally, price will be a factor in your marketing plan. You do not want to price your product/service so high that people are not willing to pay, nor should you price it too low and undervalue your product or service.

CUSTOMER SATISFACTION AND DOCUMENTATION AND EVALUATION

A satisfied customer is more likely to provide repeat business and recommend your product or service to friends and family. An unsatisfied customer may not return and can spread negative opinions about your business. In terms of business, it pays to have satisfied customers. As a business manager, you need to understand what the customer expects (quality service, quality food, etc.) and then you must meet or exceed those customer expectations. How do you determine customer satisfaction? You ask the customer. Simply asking, "Are you satisfied with your meal?" will provide little helpful feedback. You want to know specifics about the satisfaction or dissatisfaction. How likely is the customer to return to your restaurant/café? On a scale, how would the customer rate the quality of the food? Does the customer find the surroundings comfortable and accommodating? Was the food served at a desirable temperature, or was it too cold? Were the staff members friendly and the service adequate? Customer feedback should be taken seriously, documented, and evaluated to improve the performance of the organization. Customer complaints should also be addressed and documented appropriately.

STRATEGIES AND RATIONALE

A **break-even** pricing strategy is used when the company financially breaks even on the product or service rather than making a profit. This strategy can be risky because you are making no money from the product or service, but it may also deter competition and attract customers. Management can gradually increase the price after customers are obtained.

A **revenue-generating** pricing strategy generates revenue by pricing goods or services above costs. In general, organizations want to generate revenue and make a profit. Prices may be set a little above cost, and this may result in a high-sales volume, or unique/in-demand items could be sold at a premium.

Loss-leader pricing is pricing an item below cost. This type of pricing strategy can be known as penetration pricing when a product is first entering the market. Once the product has gained market share, prices may increase. Loss-leader pricing when used to put the competition out of business may be illegal.

Media Relations

Media relations is a part of public relations, and it may be an important communication and promotional tool for your business. When you work with and establish a relationship with the media, you can get your business or event promoted. Let's suppose you are hosting a weight loss program for the community, and you want to get community support, sponsors, and participants. You might issue a press release detailing your event and purpose. You may also wish to make television interview appearances to further promote the program. In working effectively with the media, you are able to reach a massive audience.

Social Networking

Social networking may include networking directly face-to-face with people, and it may also include the use of social media. Whereas social networking used to include only charity events, business dinners, and health fairs to interact with people and promote products and services, the rise of social media has changed things significantly. Social media platforms provide an avenue to reach the masses on a constant basis. Certainly, when social media is used and managed appropriately, it can open many doors when it comes to public relations and marketing. Social media sites such as Twitter, Facebook, and Instagram offer people and businesses a platform to reach an audience. If you wish to promote an upcoming weight loss program, social media is a great option to provide program details and reminders to the public.

Campaign Development

If you have a public health message or an event you wish to promote, you must consider a campaign to get the word out to the public. Perhaps you are focusing on a behavior change such as weight loss in your community, and you are holding a series of weight loss classes and workshops as part of the program. As with any type of marketing, you want to consider who your target audience is and how you are going to reach your audience. What is your message, and what are you trying to accomplish? Would the campaign benefit from a catchy slogan? What types of media will be used to reach your audience? If you are trying to promote your campaign to an entire community, a billboard might be appropriate. In addition, flyers and pamphlets at area businesses can be useful. A dedicated website and the use of social media are additional tools to help promote your objective. A well-thought-out program campaign can help facilitate success.

Customer Service

It is not enough to promote a product or service and get people to try the product/service; a business must also provide customer service during and after the service provided or the sale of a product. We are all responsible for customer service in some capacity. If we are dietitians in a hospital setting, our customers are the patients and their families. If we are involved in a foodservice setting, the restaurant patrons are the customers. Those to whom you provide goods or services are considered the customers. Why is customer service important? In general, people want to feel valued and respected, and customer service starts with this necessary step. Beyond that, people want to receive high-quality services and products because they are paying, and that is the expectation. From a business standpoint, high-quality customer service can result in repeat business, whereas poor or lacking customer service is detrimental to the business. For a hospital, providing a patient bed is not enough; high-quality service must be provided for the patient as well.

Quality Management and Improvement

Healthcare Regulatory and Accrediting Agencies

Healthcare organizations and facilities are subject to outside regulation, oversight, and accreditation. The Centers for Medicare & Medicaid Services (CMS) falls under the Department of Health and Human Services. CMS is responsible for regulating Medicare and Medicaid. The Affordable Care Act is overseen by the Center for Consumer Information and Insurance Oversight. Often, states rely on their own departments of public health to provide state oversight for healthcare facilities. In addition, other state agencies may oversee healthcare licensure. The exact nature of the regulation may vary from state to state. It is important to be familiar with the regulations associated with the state in which you are practicing. The Joint Commission on Accreditation of Healthcare Agencies offers certification for healthcare facilities; the participation is voluntary, but many facilities strive to achieve this certification as a standard of quality. The National Committee for Quality Assurance provides accreditation for health plan insurers including health maintenance organizations and preferred provider organizations.

Productivity Analysis

Healthcare organizations, just like any business, need to be productive to maximize the use of resources. The cost of healthcare continues to increase, and controlling costs is an important consideration for organizations. One must consider the current levels of productivity and determine means to increase productivity. In healthcare, productivity is often linked to quality. The use of standards-based care or evidence-based practices has a positive benefit on outcomes.

Incorporating technology into healthcare can help to streamline processes and reduce the time spent on some tasks.

Productivity = output ÷ input, where output is the product or services produced and input is labor hours.

Program and Product Analyses

Organizations should conduct a program (or product) analysis prior to the program initiation or product release. A program analysis is important because you want the program to be successful, and you need to understand the environment that will facilitate or hinder success. Consider the factors that may help lead to success. Perhaps you have a healthy budget, volunteers, healthcare professionals, and a marketing campaign that will help drive success; these are positive resources. Also, one must consider the barriers to success. Perhaps you have a limited budget, there is an anticipated resistance to change, or you are uncertain about how to best reach your target audience. You must consider how to address these constraints to success prior to implementing the project. Inevitably, projects will have constraints and limitations, but it is best to understand them and have a plan to mitigate those constraints to help make the program a success.

Foodservice Systems

Menu Development

Menus

Patient/Resident, Commercial, and Noncommercial

A patient/resident menu may be found in an inpatient, acute care hospital setting, a skilled nursing facility (nursing home), or a rehabilitation center. A commercial menu can be found at restaurants including fast-food, full-service chain restaurants, coffee shops, and local eateries. As the name commercial implies, a commercial operation seeks to gain a profit. Noncommercial menus are found in places like schools or correctional facilities. The menu offerings may differ greatly among these places because the customer or person being served is going to be very different.

Frequently Encountered

No-choice menus give the customer/consumer no choice in entrees. A no-choice menu might be used in a noncommercial setting such as an elementary school cafeteria. School children go through the lunch line and have no choice about what is served. A no-choice menu may be a cyclical menu that rotates for some period of time (e.g., a month) and then repeats. A limited-choice menu provides some options. This type of menu might be available for hospital patients or skilled nursing facility residents. For example, the menu might include baked chicken with an option to choose either salad or green beans. A limited-choice menu provides more options to guests. A static menu does not change on a daily or weekly basis and provides adequate food choices for the repeat customer. Static menus are typically offered at restaurants. Single-use menus are used frequently for catered and special events such as weddings; the exact same menu is generally not repeated. Other types of menus include du jour, which is a special menu for the day. Restaurants frequently feature a soup du jour, which is the soup of the day. A la carte menus are popular at high-end restaurants. Rather than ordering an entrée where the price includes steak, a potato, and salad, with an a la carte menu, these items are purchased separately if desired. A table d'hote menu may include a single set menu or only very few menu choices, and there is a set price for the meal.

Aspects of the Food Service System Impacted by the Menu

Essentially, the menu impacts all aspects of the food service system. The type of menu chosen will impact the budget, facility design, equipment needs, and staffing needs. A fast-food restaurant has very different needs than a full-service, high-end restaurant. Fast-food restaurants rely on quick service; the menu must consist of meals that can be prepared with limited time. A sit-down restaurant may have fresher ingredients and more options on the menu, thus requiring more storage and a larger prep area. In addition, labor needs will be different. Because of the menu offerings and prices, a high-end restaurant should have a chef, well-trained cooks, and wait staff. A fast-food restaurant typically employs kitchen staff who do not require extensive training, including cashiers, and drive-through attendants. Instead of fryers and microwaves found in a fast-food establishment, sit-down restaurants may require more gas ranges and ovens to prepare the menu items as well as space dedicated for dish washing and storage of plates, cups, and utensils. A newer twist on the restaurant is the food truck. This portable restaurant has limited space, so menu choices need to reflect the capabilities within the food truck to make it feasible.

Master Menu

Use of a Master Menu in Food Service Operations

A master menu is, in a sense, the master plan for food options. From a master menu, most changes and modifications can be made. It serves as a guide for the operation and allows necessary alterations and substitutions. For instance, you may have chicken on your master menu. There are many options in how to cook chicken (e.g., baking, frying, or grilling,) and there are different seasonings and sauces that may be used to create variety from that one menu item. From the master menu you can create modified or therapeutic diets such as low sodium or heart healthy. Having a master menu from which to work is essential in planning and can help anticipate food and staffing needs.

Menu Planning Process

Many factors must be considered when planning a menu. A primary factor to consider during the planning process is the clientele you will be serving. The menu will differ greatly if you are a hospital food service operation serving patients as opposed to a stand-alone restaurant. Nutritional adequacy will need to be considered if you are in an operation such as a school or health care facility. Another consideration is food trends. Depending on your niche, a menu serving fried and processed foods might not appeal to the people seeking healthier dining options. Budgetary concerns also have a big impact on menu items. State-run entities may have a more limited budget than a chain restaurant. In addition, the menu makeup will impact the type and number of personnel required. You must also consider equipment and space needs for properly preparing the menu items. For example, if you have fried items on your menu, you will likely need a deep fryer. In addition, you must be able to obtain the menu items at a quality and cost that are acceptable.

Guidelines and Parameters

Aesthetics

A menu should be visually appealing because you want people to purchase your food; it is essentially a marketing tool. First, you must consider your customer when designing the menu. You would expect a menu for an inpatient hospital to be different from a menu at a retail, sit-down restaurant. The look of the menu should reflect the type of establishment. As an example, a seafood restaurant at the beach might use beachy colors and be adorned with nautical items. A high-end restaurant may present a conservative, simple menu design. In contrast, a restaurant catering to children may design a menu to be colorful and bright. It is important to know the audience/customers, and a menu should be designed to appeal to those groups. Menus should have adequate margins, ample free space, and lettering large enough to be read easily by customers with impaired vision.

Nutritional Adequacy

Not all establishments choose or are required to consider nutritional adequacy. Restaurants may not consider nutritional adequacy unless there is customer desire, or they are trying to satisfy a niche. Other entities are quite different. For example, many schools receive federal funding if they participate in the Child Nutrition Program by meeting certain nutrition standards. Operations such as hospitals, rehabilitation centers, and nursing homes have a responsibility to provide adequate nutrition. Residents or patients do not have other food choices, and meeting the nutrition requirements of these populations is essential in maintaining proper health. Another entity that must consider adequate nutrition during menu planning is the military. Meals prepared on military bases must meet minimum standards. In addition, the meals ready-to-eat (MREs) are designed for soldiers in the field. These meals must also meet certain vitamin, mineral, and energy requirements.

Depending on the people who will be served, there may or may not be a need to consider nutritional adequacy during menu development.

Cost

You must consider how much money is available to spend on food items and personnel before the menu is set. Commercial operations may have a more generous budget than noncommercial entities. A high-end steak house can typically spend more on food and staffing than a hospital food service operation. A chain restaurant expanding into a new area is likely to have a larger budget than a local start-up establishment. If there is a limited budget, items such as beef filet or lobster would not be wise. In addition, menu items that require a lot of labor will result in greater expense. Entities such as schools rely primarily on tax dollars and federal funding to purchase and provide food; the result is often a very modest budget. Hospitals and rehabilitation centers may have a per-person/patient budget, so the dollars available will vary, but the budget may be limited. Whatever the type of food service operation, the menu must reflect the resources available.

Regulations

Regulations dictate that menus be truthful; you cannot misrepresent a food item or make misleading statements. These regulations are commonly known as the truth in menu laws. For instance, if you are a food service operation in Florida, and on the menu, you state the corn is locally grown, that claim is untruthful if the corn is actually grown in Nebraska. If the menu indicates you are serving Kobe beef, the beef must be from a certain type of cattle, or you cannot make that claim. A menu item listing a dessert with fresh strawberries must include fresh strawberries, not frozen. If a health claim on a menu is made, the claim should have validity. In addition to truthful labeling, a regulation from the Food and Drug Administration that is set to go into effect in 2018 will require calorie information to be listed on menus. At present, this rule applies to large chain restaurants with twenty or more locations. During menu development, it is essential to be aware of any federal, state, or local regulations dealing with food service and menu labeling.

Modifications

Diet/Disease States/Lifespan

Modified Diets in a Hospital Food Service Setting

Depending on the facility, the diet name may vary slightly, but inpatient facilities have modified or therapeutic diets to meet the medical or dietary needs of patients. Examples of modified diets include the following:

- A clear liquid diet consists of liquids that are clear, such as fruit juice, tea, and broth. A clear liquid diet should not continue for more than forty-eight hours because it does not provide enough nutrients.
- A full liquid diet tends to be a more substantial and includes milk, ice cream, and pudding. If a full liquid diet is ordered for more than a few days, nutritional adequacy must be evaluated.
- A mechanical soft diet may be ordered for someone who has poor dentition or difficulty properly chewing.
- Other modified diets include low sodium, low fiber, cardiac prudent/heart healthy, diabetic, dysphagia, and renal.

In addition to addressing the disease state, one must always consider the nutritional adequacy of the diet. Modified diets can be altered from the master menu by following the instructions in the facility's diet manual.

Dysphagia Diet

A dysphagia diet is ordered when a patient has swallowing difficulties. This is very common in post-stroke patients. After a consult with the speech therapist, the degree of swallowing difficulty is determined. Depending on necessity, a diet consisting of pureed foods may be ordered. The foods are blended or pureed to achieve a very soft, wet consistency. This aids in safe swallowing. A less restrictive dysphagia diet may be ordered if swallowing is less impaired. Foods in this category have a more solid consistency and may include ground meat and chopped food items. The goal of the dysphagia diet is to progress to a diet with regular consistency.

Cardiac Prudent Diet

A cardiac prudent or heart healthy diet may be ordered for patients hospitalized due to a heart attack or underlying heart disease. A heart healthy diet will place limits on sodium intake and saturated fat. Depending on the facility guidelines, cholesterol and total fat may also be limited. A good example of a cardiac diet meal is baked chicken, a garden salad, whole grain pasta, and a side of fruit. Care should be taken to limit high-sodium items, which may be found in canned goods and seasonings. Meats that are high in saturated fat such as some beef and pork products should not be offered on the heart healthy diet.

Substitutions

From time to time, there may be a need to deviate from the master menu. Perhaps there is an issue with the supplier and the product is no longer available, or the price has increased dramatically due to low supply. It is also possible the restaurant or facility runs out of an item and must substitute a comparable item on a short-term basis. Customer request may also dictate the need for substitutions. Whether it is simply a food preference, a cultural or religious preference, or food allergy, an operation should be prepared to substitute roughly equivalent items when necessary.

Common Food Allergies and Sensitivities

Although the vast majority of customers do not suffer from a food allergy, it is a good business practice to provide options for those who do. Certainly, not every restaurant can address every food allergy. Some restaurants, upon introduction of the server, will inquire about any food allergies or sensitivities. Frequently the chef will accommodate these types of special requests by altering the menu. Common food allergies include peanut/tree nut, seafood/shellfish, wheat, egg, milk/soy, and gluten. Although not a true allergy, some people are believed to be sensitive to gluten. Several restaurants now offer gluten-free items that are similar to their regular menu offerings, such as gluten-free pizza. A balanced menu, by offering variety, can help address some food allergies. For instance, many restaurants offer a combination of steak, chicken, and seafood. This provides many options for someone who is allergic to seafood or shellfish. Nut-free desserts are another example of a menu modification that caters to allergy sufferers. For breakfast fare, menus may offer egg substitutes. Although it is unrealistic to create a menu to address all food allergies, it is important to be knowledgeable about allergies and, when possible, work with the customer to provide alternatives.

Cultural/Religious

It is important to be aware and sensitive to cultural and religious food preferences. Some religions may have strict laws about what should and should not be eaten. Jewish people follow a kosher diet, and there are some restrictions about what can be eaten and how the food is prepared. Jewish people do not eat pork, which includes hotdogs and bacon. In addition, shellfish is not acceptable, but beef, chicken, duck, goose, and turkey are permitted. In general, fruits and vegetables are considered acceptable. It is also not permitted to eat meat and milk together, so this should be noted in meal planning. In addition, certain food ingredients are not considered kosher, and these common ingredients include gelatin, casein, lard, and shortening.

Vegetarian/Vegan

There are many reasons one may need to alter the master menu. If in a hospital or skilled nursing facility setting, modified therapeutic diets may be ordered. Examples of such diets include heart healthy, low sodium, and low fiber. In addition, master menus may be altered to accommodate vegetarian preferences. In place of a meat, a vegetable or soy-based protein may be substituted. Also, there may be cultural or religious preferences one must consider. In addition, the menu may be altered due to an item's lack of availability or seasonality. For example, during the summer months fresh fruits or vegetables may be added to the menu.

Satisfaction Indicators

Customer Evaluation and Sales Data

Whether you are just opening a business, expanding or adding new menu items, or are an established operation, customer satisfaction is important. If you are in a commercial operation such as a restaurant, a good indicator of menu satisfaction is steady and repeat business. One way to observe repeat business is through analyzing sales trends and data. Take a period of time, a month for example, and divide total sales (in dollars) by the number of customers. If the number seems lower than normal, this may indicate menu dissatisfaction. Another method to evaluate satisfaction is through the use of surveys. Surveys may ask about the likability of an item or may inquire about how frequently the customer might be willing to order the menu item (i.e., every visit, on occasion, or never). In hospital and residential settings (nursing homes), plate waste is often a good indicator of satisfaction. Plate waste is assessed simply by looking at the amount of food left uneaten.

Operational Influences

Equipment

As the menu is being developed, it is important to consider the type of equipment needed to prepare and store food items. The food items on the menu will dictate the type of equipment needed to properly prepare the items. A fast-food operation and sandwich shop will have different equipment needs than a full-service, sit-down restaurant. In turn, a hospital serving hundreds of patients three meals daily will have different equipment needs than a commercial restaurant. A fast-food operation will require equipment aimed at quick preparation and service. Thus, you might expect deep fryers, griddles, and warmers. A sandwich shop may require meat slicers and ovens for baking bread. A full-service, sit down restaurant may offer a more expanded menu and will likely require more varied equipment. The needs of a full-service restaurant will likely include gas ranges, griddles or grills, ovens, steam kettles, frying pans, mixers, and dishwashing machines. A hospital is likely serving three meals a day plus snacks. Given the large volume served, equipment will need to address this need. Depending on the menu, food storage needs must also be assessed. Ample refrigeration space will be needed for fresh meats and produce, whereas freezer storage will need to accommodate frozen items.

Labor

When deciding on a menu, you must consider labor needs. Consider the type of food service establishment and the staff you can afford to hire. Determine the types of skills the workers must possess and the availability of this skill sets. If you have $46 filets on the menu, customers will expect good wait staff, skilled cooks, and a chef. If you plan to offer pastries, a qualified pastry chef is necessary. On the contrary, if you own a sandwich shop, the skill sets will be quite different. The staff needed may take orders and put together sandwiches, which require fewer skills, less labor, and a smaller labor budget. So, when you decide on menu items, it is necessary to consider whether or not you can staff the operation to deliver the quality and service desired.

External Influences

Seasonality

Seasonality can play a role in the food preferences of the customer and also the products available for purchase by the food service operation. For instance, it may be more difficult to acquire fresh vegetables in the winter months versus the summer. If you do wish to acquire these fresh products, they are likely to be more expensive, and quality may be diminished because they will need to be brought in from a distance. In addition, customers often prefer different foods in the winter. A hot cup of soup or a pot roast is more appealing in cooler weather versus the hot summer months. Likewise, a fresh dinner salad or cool, refreshing specialty fruit drink is often more desirable in the summer. Because of these reasons, restaurants and other food service operations may alter their menus somewhat based on the seasons.

Emergency Management

Depending on the type of operation, the menu for emergency management will differ. Commercial restaurants will likely close during an emergency and would not need an emergency menu. Other organizations such as hospitals or college dining halls will need to stay open and should have emergency menus in place to serve patients or customers for a period of time. If the event is expected—for example, a hurricane is expected, and widespread power outages and flooding is predicted—you have time prepare and order extra stock. Large-scale operations typically have a backup power generator to power systems in case of power outages, so kitchens may be able to serve hot meals and operate at near-normal capacity. During an emergency, labor shortages may occur, so the menu should be labor and resource sparing if possible, to limit the fatigue on power generators. In the event of a complete power outage, there should be a stockpile of shelf-stable items. The stockpile may include bottled water, cereals, peanut butter, crackers, canned fruit and vegetables, canned meats, fruit juices, and cereal bars. Manual can openers and disposable plates and utensils should also be available.

Procurement, Production, Distribution, and Service

Procurement Principles, Concepts, and Methods

Bid Process and Contract Implementation

Competitive bidding involves putting out a request for a proposal (RFP) for food items. Food vendors may then bid on the proposal by providing food prices, food specifications, and other terms the proposal may have detailed. Food specifications will be important because it describes or specifies the food needs and requirements. Food specs detail size, quantity, quality, grade, brand, and so on. Detailed specifications help ensure you get what you want and decrease ambiguity. After the proposal window has closed, all bids are evaluated based on the criteria set forth. Competitive bidding may help an organization get the lowest prices for the best products. Government organizations are often required to use this type of bidding process. An alternative to the competitive bid process is open market bidding. This process is simpler and less time-consuming than the competitive bid process. The purchaser simply orders the food and quantities needed based on the quoted prices from vendors. A purchaser may use several different suppliers or change to a supplier that offers a better price, better quality, or better service. Typically, smaller food service operations will use the informal approach.

Specification Development

In addition to product names and quantities, food specs need to be very detailed so the product you receive is the product you expected. Food grade should be specified so that when you want prime beef to serve your customers, you receive the top quality cut you are expecting instead of choice or select grades. When ordering fresh vegetables and fruits, desirable qualities should be noted such as firm, bright green, or red. With the purchase of canned goods, the purchaser should indicate details such as canned in own juices, whole green beans, cut green beans, or whole kernel corn. The size (e.g., no. 10 can) and count per container should also be specified. The fat content of dairy products needs to be listed because dairy products may be classified as whole, low-fat, or skim.

Group Purchasing/Prime Vendor

Group purchasing involves several different entities joining together to make purchases. The primary advantage of this is decreased food prices because of increased order volume. In group purchasing, the entities are not related. This differs from centralized purchasing in which the facilities are related. For example, the central office at a county school district may purchase all foods for the entire district rather than each school purchasing independently. A prime vendor is one who is selected to provide the majority of food items or products for the restaurant or organization. Because the vendor has an exclusive contract for a specified period of time, there is likely a financial advantage offered to the buyer.

Ethics

The relationship between the buyer and vendor must remain a professional one in appearance and in reality. Although this relationship may be friendly in nature, a buyer should never accept gifts from a vendor. Accepting a gift may be seen as a bribe to ensure the continuation of a purchasing agreement even if the gift is innocent or seemingly only a kind gesture. A gift in exchange for continued business is unethical; purchasing should be made based on business needs and cost rather than a self-serving agreement. The buyer must always consider the needs of his/her organization and make decisions accordingly.

Procurement Decisions

Product Selection/Yield, Product Packaging, and Cost Analysis

Food preparation time, costs, and storage concerns may influence purchasing decisions. Frozen foods require ample freezer space but may be kept longer than fresh foods and result in less waste or spoilage. In addition, purchasing bulk packages will be less expensive but requires more storage space. Although bulk purchasing is more economical, it becomes less so if it results in foods waste because the quantity may exceed actual needs. Fresh meats and vegetables require refrigerated storage, and adequate space must be available. Fresh fruits and vegetables also tend to be quite expensive, so the budget is a factor. The decision to purchase whole versus sliced food products may also be impacted by budget and time. Pre-sliced foods can save on labor time in the prep area. Whole fruits and vegetables may require cutting, slicing, or peeling. Also, one must consider customer preference and expectations. When patronizing certain restaurants, the customer may expect freshly prepared foods. When deciding upon food form, it is important to consider costs, storage, labor, and customer expectations.

Receiving and Storage

Receiving Procedures for a Food Shipment

Receiving an order involves comparing the ordered items to the items received. You want to make sure you received what you are expecting at the agreed-upon prices. An invoice should accompany each order and should list the items and prices. One may check the items against the original purchase order before accepting, or the receiver may inspect and count each individual item—this is known as the blind check method. Equipment may be needed to move and open delivery items. If the deliveries are large, a forklift may be needed. Hand carts can be used to move smaller items, and box cutters may be needed to easily open boxes. Upon arrival, a thermometer should be available to check temperatures of items requiring refrigeration. Refrigerated foods should be kept below 40°F. Also, frozen foods should be inspected to ensure they have been properly transported and are still frozen. Improper temperatures of foods pose a safety risk. Any problems or discrepancies with the order should be documented and a record kept of receipts. Received items should be moved to their designated storage areas as soon as possible. This is especially urgent for items that need refrigeration or freezers. The receiving area must be kept safe and secure; quick removal of items from the delivery dock helps minimize the threat of theft or tampering.

Food Storage

The main types of storage in a food service operation are dry storage, refrigerated, and freezer storage. Foods and supplies that do not need to be refrigerated or frozen belong in dry storage. To maintain an optimal environment for the food, the area must be well-ventilated and cool, and humidity should be controlled. Items should never be placed directly on the floor or against the wall. Items should be rearranged with the oldest items in the front and the newest items in the back. This process is known as first in first out (FIFO). Following this method helps ensure the older items will be used first; thus, the operation has less food waste from food going stale or being out of date. Refrigerators are used to store items that are typically held at 40°F or below. Optimal temperatures do vary for some refrigerated products, and ideally an operation has a separate refrigerator to accommodate. Fresh vegetables and fruits should be held at 40 to 45°F. Dairy, eggs, and meat products should be held between 32 and 40°F. Frozen foods are kept in the freezer, and temperatures are held between 0 and –10°F. Thermometers should be in place to monitor temperature.

Inventory Management

Inventory management should follow a fairly formal process to ensure effectiveness. Just as items received should be signed in or recorded, items removed from inventory must be authorized, and the item(s) removed should be recorded. To request food or supplies, a requisition form is used; a requisition aids in inventory control. It is essential to track the items one currently has in inventory and the items that have been removed; a proper system helps with cost control. Technology has simplified and streamlined the process of inventory management, but the use of technology varies depending on the operation. A record of items used, items currently in storage, and items removed is known as the perpetual inventory. Minimum or maximum inventory amounts should be established by the food service operation. When a product falls below par level (minimum level allowed), the item should be reordered. The maximum level includes items needed for use plus some extra in case an unusual situation arises.

Benefit of Technology

A comprehensive inventory management system can provide the food service manager with constant, up-to-date information. Technology is more accurate, saves time, and can save money. Operations typically have a lot of money tied up in inventory, and the better inventory is managed, the better the finances of the organization. Technology can help track items in multiple inventory locations, which saves time. With technology, it is easy to view how much of an item is in storage, where it is located, and when it will need to be reordered. With effective uses of technology, a facility is less likely to have excess inventory on hand, resulting in food waste, and less likely to run below par level or out of an item completely. Technology can also assist with invoicing, reordering, and valuing inventory.

Inventory Scenario

You are getting ready to prepare a meal for a big banquet. You notice you are low on flour even though the inventory sheet indicates you have plenty. Explain what may have happened.

> It is likely flour was removed from inventory, and the proper procedures were not followed. It is possible a requisition form was not completed by the staff needing the flour, and the flour was removed without permission. The supply room may have been left unlocked allowing uncontrolled access. It is possible the item was not recorded or tracked at the time of removal by the supply manager. Perhaps someone intended to record the removal at a later time and ultimately failed or forgot to document it. It is essential to follow proper inventory management procedures each and every time to avoid supply shortages or excess. It may be necessary to physically count inventory from time to time to ensure the items listed in inventory reflect what is actually available.

Cooking Methods

Dispersion

A dispersion is a mixture of substances. The art of food preparation and cooking is about mixing ingredients in the right amounts to produce a desirable product. A dispersion is classified by the state of matter (solid, liquid, or gas) and the particle size. For example, mayonnaise represents a liquid in liquid dispersion and a sponge cake is an example of a gas in solid dispersion. A true solution is a dispersion containing the smallest particles. Salt completely dissolves in water and is a true solution. Colloidal dispersions contain medium-sized particles, and jelly is an example of colloidal dispersion. A specific type of colloidal dispersion is known as an emulsion; an emulsion is a dispersion of two liquids. Mayonnaise is a common example of an oil-in-water emulsion. Butter is a water-in-oil emulsion. Dispersions can be changed in a variety of ways such applying heat (cooking) and freezing.

Functions of Acid in Cooking

The acid content of food affects the ability of pathogens to grow and reproduce. Foods with a higher acid content (lower pH) are not as susceptible to microorganism growth. Vegetables tend to have a higher pH and must be processed and canned at a temperature above 212°F to destroy botulinum. To freeze vegetables, they should be blanched first (submersion in boiling followed by ice water). Fruits have a higher acid content and are less susceptible to microbial growth. Preservation of fruits does not require extreme heat; it is appropriate to wash and freeze rather than blanching first. In addition to affecting microbial growth, acids also play a role in food appearance. Because acids are released during the cooking process, vegetables that have been cooked too long or canned may lose their bright colors. Canned green beans are an example of vegetables that show color loss; instead of a green color, they may appear browner in color.

Equipment

The type of equipment used in cooking will affect the cooking process, the speed of cooking, and the quality of the final product. Baking pans, dishes, and skillets conduct heat according to their consistency. For example, copper and iron skillets tend to be good conductors of heat, whereas glass is a poor conductor. Ovens are used to transfer heat in an enclosed space; a convection oven differs from a conventional oven in that air is circulated with a fan. The advantage with convection is faster cooking time because heat is transferred more readily. A convection oven may be used for meats to decrease the baking time while maintaining flavor and moisture. Heat radiation does not rely on food coming into direct contact with the heat source; the use of a microwave is s a good example of radiant heat. Microwave heating tends to be inconsistent in that heating may be uneven in the food product. In practice, cooking is often a combination of conduction, convection, and radiation heat transfer.

Food Preservation and Packing Methods

The first priority in food preservation is safety, so killing the majority of microorganisms present prior to preserving is essential. Freezing is a common method of food preservation; freezing can destroy or significantly slow the growth of microorganisms. Vegetables should be blanched before freezing to eliminate microbes and help maintain color. Commercially frozen vegetables may be packaged in plastic bags. Fruit is too delicate to blanch, and the acid content in fruit helps prevent microbial growth. Fruit may be washed then frozen in plastic bags to preserve and store. Food drying or dehydrating reduces the water content and is another form of food preservation. Because the moisture content is low, microbial growth is limited. Meats like beef jerky and dried fruits are examples of dehydrated foods. Canning is a food preservation and packing method that uses high heat to kill microorganisms. Canned foods are shelf stable for a long period of time. Freeze drying and vacuum packaging are additional ways to preserve and package foods. Freeze drying involves first freezing the food and then removing the moisture. Vacuum packaging removes a majority of the oxygen from the package, which inhibits the growth of microorganisms.

Modified Food Preparation

Genetically modified foods continue to be controversial even though they have been around for many years. Genetically modified foods are common and include corn, soybeans, and zucchini. A genetically modified food is one in which the DNA has been changed by processes that do not occur in nature. The DNA has been modified in such a way to present a desired outcome, but there are concerns modifications will produce unintended or unknown consequences. Benefits of genetic engineering may include nutrient density, increased crop production, and lower costs. Concerns about genetically modified foods come from a lack of understanding and lack of proven safety. Although the regulation has yet to take effect, in 2016 Congress passed a law requiring genetically modified foods to be identified by labeling.

Standardized Recipes and Ingredient Control

Standardizing recipes help ensure food quality and consistency regardless of who is preparing the food. Most food service organizations employ many kitchen staff, and employee turnover is common. Regardless of whether a veteran cook is working or a new employee, standardized recipes should help ensure a consistent meal every time. Chain restaurants use standardized recipes, and whether you go to Restaurant X in Florida or California, the menu items should taste very similar if the recipe is followed properly. A standardized recipe has clear directions and is adapted to the specific needs of the food service organization; a quality product is expected with each production. A standardized recipe also helps in forecasting, ingredient control, and overall cost control. Ingredients, ingredient amounts, product yield, and specific, step by step directions are detailed on the recipe; any variations of the recipe are also noted.

Portion Control and Yield Analysis

In a large-scale food service operation, it is essential to anticipate the product yield and to control portions. You need to make enough food for the customers, but you do not want to make too much, which results in food waste. Although some food waste is expected, it should be minimized to help control costs. The standardized recipe indicates the expected yield of a product, and portion size must be noted when serving. Suppose you make four pans of lasagna, and each pan is expected serve 25 portions for a total of 100 servings. However, upon plating the lasagna the actual yield is 85 servings. Either the recipe did not yield the expected number of servings or the incorrect portions were served. Perhaps instead of serving the 3x5-inch pieces of lasagna, someone accidentally served 4x5-inch portions. The result is not enough food for the dinner meal. Any discrepancies in product yield must be noted and evaluated.

Forecasting Production

Forecasting is an attempt to anticipate what is going to happen. Food service operations attempt to plan ahead to minimize shortfalls in food and staffing. For instance, a restaurant should know the number of customers and meals typically served in a day along with menu items that are most popular. With the information, food and supply orders are placed, and employee schedules are made. If you are unable to forecast accurately, the operation may run out of food, which displeases the customer. On the flip side, the restaurant may procure too much or prepare an excess of the product; this results in food waste. Forecasting methods may vary depending on the operation. A popular method to aid in forecasting is using historical data. This approach is straightforward and uses data from the past to help predict the future. This method works well when there are not many fluctuations in day-to-day or week-to-week business. Computer modeling methods help can help forecast with greater accuracy and may account for seasonality or other influences.

Production Scheduling

Production planning is key to success in any food service operation; this planning step is especially pivotal in large-scale operations. Kitchen staff must know what food items to prepare, when to prepare, the quantity needed, who is tasked with preparation and cooking, and completion times for each task. For example, suppose you manage food service for a 900-bed hospital, and breakfast service begins at 7:00 am followed by lunch at 11:00 am. Production must have a detailed schedule and know their assigned tasks to produce the meal in an efficient manner. Timing is essential; you do not want to have the food ready too early because quality and food safety and are compromised. In addition, you do not want to run behind in production because the result is late tray delivery.

Delayed service impacts the production schedule for the rest of the day and may cause customer dissatisfaction.

Production Systems

Conventional

A conventional food service system is one in which food is prepared and served in the same location. For example, most restaurants are considered conventional operations. The food is prepared on site in the kitchen and typically delivered to the patron in the dining area. Restaurants, schools, and hospitals typically use the conventional system. This system allows for foods to be delivered shortly after preparation to ensure maximum quality and provides more flexibility in food choices than other production systems. Typically, this type of production system is labor intensive.

Commissary

A commissary production system is where food is purchased and prepared in a central location and then transported to other unit locations. This type of operation may be found in large schools or hospital systems. Food produced may be frozen, chilled, or held hot prior to transport. A centralized production area helps contain the costs of having multiple kitchen facilities and production staff. The disadvantages to this process are delivery challenges, logistics, and concerns with food safety. Foods must be kept at safe temperatures and not allowed to fall into danger zones.

Other Production Systems

A ready-prepared system is one where food is prepared on site and held for use later. Depending on the length of time between preparation and service (often several days), the food may be frozen or chilled. The ready-prepared system differs from the commissary system in that food is not served immediately, but it is served on site. An assembly-serve system is one with no on-site food production. Prepared foods are purchased, and the facility needs only to assemble (if required), heat, and serve. The cook-chill method involves cooking food items and very quickly chilling the items using a blast chiller for use at a later date. Display cooking, as the name implies, is where you can see the food being prepared. This type involves the senses (see, hear, and smell the foods) and has become quite popular in recent years. Typically, the food prep is completed in advance, and the food is cooked in front of the customer. Display cooking may involve permanent, built-in display units, or the display unit may be temporary and transportable.

Type of Service Systems

Centralized delivery is common in hospital food service settings. Food is placed on trays in a central location such as the kitchen, and the trays are transported to the customer/patient. Heated and refrigerated carts or insulated trays may be used to maintain food temperature during the delivery process. Decentralized delivery is where food is prepared in the kitchen and transported to the customer/patient area prior to plating. This type of setup may be used when there is a significant distance between the kitchen and the customer. Once the food carts arrive on location, food may be reheated, plated, and then delivered to the customer. Given the travel distance from kitchen to customer, this option may provide a more desirable product (maintain proper temperature) than central plating. Decentralized delivery tends to be more expensive because it is labor intensive and typically requires duplication of equipment among the units.

Equipment and Packaging

In a commissary production system especially, transportation from one physical location to another provides challenges in terms of food safety and food quality. The type of equipment used and the food packaging help mitigate many problems. Mobile pans with lids are often used both for cooking and transportation; this alleviates the need to transfer the food to another container. Whether items are hot or frozen, insulated carriers are used to help maintain the proper food temperature during transportation. Items are then placed into trucks for timely delivery to the designated facilities. Regardless of the service/production system used, maintaining food quality and safety is essential. Facilities frequently use insulated trays, insulated plates, insulated carts, and mobile refrigeration to achieve the desired outcome. The type of equipment used depends on the individual needs of the food service organization.

Sanitation and Safety

SANITATION

SANITATION PRACTICES AND INFECTION CONTROL

PERSONAL HYGIENE

Proper hygiene and food safety begins with adequate training of the food service worker. Continuing education among food service staff along with specific policies and procedures addressing sanitation and cleanliness should be communicated. Staff must dress appropriately in either a uniform or clean, washable clothing. Hair restraints/hair nets should be worn to cover head and facial hair; this prevents hair from coming into contact with food. Jewelry, especially rings and watches, should not be worn because they may harbor bacteria that can be transferred to food. Additional hygiene measures include the following:

- Short, trimmed fingernails
- Disposable gloves used when directly handling food
- Smoking allowed only in designated areas
- Cuts or opens sores properly covered with a waterproof bandage
- Sick workers remaining home
- Proper handwashing procedures

FOOD AND EQUIPMENT

Work surfaces and anything that comes into contact with food must be cleaned and sanitized. Work surfaces may include cutting boards, pans, plates, spoons, or any other equipment. Depending on the equipment, some appliances must be completely disassembled to adequately clean, whereas other types of equipment require little or no disassembly. Equipment that is used continuously must be cleaned and sanitized several times a day.

Cleaning involves using some type of cleaning agent such as detergent to scrub the surface followed by rinsing to remove any excess debris. After cleaning, the surface must be sanitized. Sanitizing is done by using a heat or a chemical agent. If using heat, the recommended temperature should reach between 162°F and 165°F. Chemical sanitizing involves submerging the item in a sanitizing solution for a period of time or spraying a chemical solution onto the object.

WASTE DISPOSAL AND FOOD HANDLING TECHNIQUES

Proper handwashing technique is essential to help prevent the spread of disease. The following procedures should be used:

1. Use warm water to wet hands.
2. Apply soap.
3. Scrub thoroughly for at least 20 seconds, being careful to scrub wrists, forearms, and between fingers.
4. Scrub tips of fingers and nails.
5. While continuing to rub hands together, rinse with warm water.
6. Dry hands using a paper towel.
7. If necessary, use a paper towel to turn off the faucet; do not recontaminate hands by touching surfaces.

Handwashing should occur in the following circumstances or as often as necessary:

- After the food service worker comes into contact with body fluids (such as going to the restroom)
- Before starting work or after a break
- After coughing or sneezing
- After eating or drinking
- After smoking or smokeless tobacco use
- Following the handling of raw food
- After touching dirty dishes or equipment
- Before food preparation

Food Laws and Regulations

The Food Safety and Inspection Service (FSIS) falls under the United States Department of Agriculture (USDA) umbrella of agencies. The FSIS is responsible for ensuring meat, poultry, and eggs are safe. The Centers for Disease Control (CDC) provide surveillance for food-borne illness outbreaks. The Food and Drug Administration (FDA) is responsible for regulating safety of food products other than meat, poultry, and eggs. An FDA regulation known as Generally Recognized as Safe (GRAS) says a food additive is subject to testing unless it has been deemed safe after long-term use. In other words, the additive has been around for so long without posing a danger that the safety of the additive is generally agreed upon. The Delaney Clause states food additives known to cause cancer are not permitted for use. The FDA also provides protection against unfair labeling practices. At the state level, state departments of public health carry out the role of investigating food-borne illnesses and inspecting food service operations.

Food Safety

Principles

Contamination and Spoilage

According to the CDC, the most common risk factors linked to food-borne illness are as follows:

- Purchase of food from an unreliable or unsafe source (it is important to know vendors and food sources)
- Food cooked incorrectly (chicken not cooked to the proper temperature poses risks for salmonella; hamburgers not fully cooked may harbor E. coli)
- Foods held at incorrect temperatures (40°F–140°F is known as the danger zone)
- Equipment contamination (cutting board used for cutting raw chicken not cleaned or sanitized then used to chop raw vegetables)
- Poor personal hygiene among food handlers (lack of proper hand washing, etc.)

Microbiological Control

Ultimately, the food service manager is responsible for food safety in his/her establishment. Managers must be well-educated about food safety, and they must properly and continuously train employees on the dangers of food-borne illness. Managers are responsible for knowing and following all laws pertaining to food safety. The manager must understand the dangers of equipment cross-contamination as well contamination by food handlers. Food handlers known to have a medical issue that may cause a food-borne illness must not be permitted to work until cleared by a doctor. Personal hygiene must be stressed and enforced in the organization. The manager is responsible for ensuring equipment is properly cleaned, sanitized, and maintained because cross-contamination is often a source of illness. He/she must understand the importance of proper food handling, storage, and cooking and ensure these procedures are followed. He/she should be well versed in time and temperature control measures because some foods such as sprouts and cut melons are more likely to support microbial growth. The food service manager must understand all aspects of food safety and implement procedures to facilitate a safe environment.

Signs and Symptoms of Food Borne Illness

Common pathogens that cause food-borne illnesses in the U.S.:

1. Salmonella is a bacterium commonly found in chicken and egg products. Symptoms include gastrointestinal upset, diarrhea, vomiting, and fever.
2. Listeria monocytogenes is a bacterium found in deli meats, soft cheeses, and unpasteurized dairy products. Symptoms include pregnancy miscarriage and meningitis in newborns.
3. The norovirus is a virus found in shellfish from contaminated water. The norovirus causes gastrointestinal problems such as vomiting, diarrhea, and cramping.
4. Campylobacter is caused by a bacterium often found in poultry, contaminated water, stews, and gravies. Symptoms include headache, fever, cramping, vomiting, and diarrhea.
5. Clostridium perfringens is a bacterium that produces toxins once ingested. It is found in foods such as meat, poultry, and stews. Diarrhea and abdominal pain are common symptoms.
6. E. coli is a bacterium that produces toxins after ingestion. Ground beef and contaminated vegetables and fruits are common sources. Diarrhea and cramping are common; kidney failure may result in severe cases.

Food Safety Management

HACCP

HACCP stands for hazard analysis critical control point. HACCP is a means of addressing food safety from all points on the food service/production continuum. The primary focus is prevention of food-borne illness and other food hazards, but simply implementing HACCP alone will not address all problems. HACCP is intended to be used along with other food safety protocol, not as a stand-alone program. Continued education and monitoring of performance must also be part of the process. HACCP has become the industry standard in terms of food safety programs and if properly implemented can help deter problems. The HACCP plan is based on seven principles:

1. Analyze and identify potential hazards that may cause sickness or harm.
2. Know critical control points (CCPs) for foods—a CCP is where/when a potential problem may arise.
3. Identify critical limits for control points.
4. Determine how to monitor CCPs.
5. Develop a corrective action plan.
6. Determine if the system is working.
7. Maintain appropriate records or documentation.

Time and Temperature Control

The food danger zone is between 40°F and 140°F. In this range, conditions are right for rapid microbial growth. The time a food is exposed to the danger zone should be minimized because the longer the food is in the zone, the more potential for microbial growth. Cold foods should maintain a temperature of less than 40°F, and hot foods should be held above 140°F. Monitoring food temperature throughout each step of the food service process is essential. Temperature must be checked upon delivery arrival, refrigerators and freezers should have thermometers, and temperature must be monitored during food production and holding. Food should never be left out to cool and later refrigerated. The time to properly cool at room temperature may take hours, exposing the food to the danger zone. Food must be cooled quickly by transferring to small, shallow containers and refrigerating immediately. According to the Food and Drug Administration Food Code, foods should be cooled to 70°F within two hours and from 70°F to 41°F or less within a four-hour period.

Documentation/Record Keeping and Recalls

Foods are typically recalled for safety reasons; the product may be mislabeled, or it may be known or suspected to contain a pathogen or foreign object. If a food product has been mislabeled, this may pose a danger to individuals with food allergies. Other products may contain foreign bodies such as glass or metal, possibly generated from the production process. Foods may also be contaminated with microorganisms such as E. coli or listeria. Prompt action regarding recalls is necessary to minimize the effects. Once a recall notification is received, the recall must be communicated throughout the organization; this communication should include any satellite sites. It must be determined and documented whether any recalled food has been served to the public. Communication to the public will be necessary if the product poses a health risk and has been served. The recalled product should be located in storage, specifically identified, and counted. Recalled food should be removed from storage and placed in an alternate location with a notice relaying the recall and a "Do Not Use" message. At this point, there should be specific instructions from the food manufacturer about how to proceed to return or destroy the product and receive a refund. It is essential to document the recall steps taken and all communications by the organization in the recall process.

Operational Emergencies

Challenges - The first step in dealing with an emergency is to be prepared. Each food service operation should have a plan tailored to the specifics of the operation and community served. Natural disasters like floods, hurricanes, and tornados can bring catastrophic results. A food service operation may have large backup generators to maintain power, but depending on the emergency, generators may fail. Hurricanes may produce wind damage and flooding. If flooding is expecting, try to minimize the damage by moving stored food to a higher location. If flood waters come into contact with food and supplies, they must be discarded. If possible, freeze refrigerated foods so they may be salvaged. If power is completely lost, keep freezers and refrigerator doors closed to maintain temperature for a short period of time. For a prolonged outage, temperatures will not be maintained, and food is no longer safe to consume; it must be discarded. Some operations such as hospitals must maintain services even during an emergency, and these operations will need to have a stockpile of nonperishable food items. If the emergency situation is ongoing, and there is a complete loss of power, adequate food supply, sufficient labor availability, proper food storage (lack of refrigeration or freezers), and inability to cook will pose a serious threat.

Organizations That Provide Food - Several entities may be involved in disaster response, but most notable are the American Red Cross and Federal Emergency Management Agency. Together, they are most responsible for setting up shelters and providing emergency food at various locations. The Red Cross coordinates with other organizations and faith-based entities to provide the needed resources. In serious emergency situations, feeding on a large scale will be needed. Central feeding and shelter sites may be set up at churches and schools, but other feeding sites may need to be established. Additional locations may be set up to provide food and clean water for first responders, high-risk groups in affected communities, and others who are unable to seek shelter.

Bioterrorism

Bioterrorism may occur in many forms, but one avenue is through the food supply. Unlike a food-borne illness, bioterrorism involves intentional tampering with the intent to create harm. Preventative measures and training known as food defense is becoming increasingly important as threats increase. Food service operations should review emergency protocols, and food defense must be assessed and addressed through education and planning. Both management and employees should understand and be prepared to address the threats posed. The primary focus of food defense is to prevent an attack. Knowing where the food has been and who will have contact with the food is vital. Prompt removal of food from loading dock and limited access to food storage areas are key components of maintaining a safe food supply. If an attack on the food supply occurs, a plan should be in place to address the attack and minimize harm. Finally, have a communication plan in place to contact anyone affected by the tainted food.

Safety

Employee

Equipment Use and Maintenance

Although it is important to protect the consumer from risk, it is also important to provide safety for food service employees. Proper use and maintenance of equipment helps reduce accidents. Food service staff must be educated about proper safety protocols not only at hiring but throughout the employment tenure. All equipment must be cleaned and maintained in proper working order, and records should be kept of all maintenance procedures. Given the circumstances, fires are a major risk in the kitchen. Equipment and lines should be periodically inspected for gas leaks and exposed wiring, and employees should take care when cooking over an open flame. Burns are another common occurrence, and employees must be cautious when handling hot pans and steamers. The use of knives and other sharp devices in the food service operation contributes to cuts and abrasions. Employees should be instructed in proper knife use, and knives should be stored when not in use. Other equipment such as slicers and can openers should be covered and stored when not in use and inspected periodically to ensure proper working order.

Personal Work Habits

The safety of employees relies on training and employees following the rules. Any unsafe working condition and accidents should be reported to the manager to prevent ongoing problems. Precautions can be taken to limit accidents in the food service establishment. Falls are common accidents that are often preventable by walking rather than running; horseplay is unacceptable and contributes to unsafe conditions. Water, grease, and food spills are common and should be cleaned up immediately to prevent falling. Aisles should be clutter free to limit tripping hazards. Proper attire is expected including close-toed shoes that provide some traction and support. Clothing should not hang down or drag on the floor. Very loose clothing may contribute to falls and could catch on fire if near an open flame. Proper lifting procedures should be followed to prevent back injury.

Practices

Environmental Conditions and Regulations

The Occupational Safety and Health Act is a law that dictates safe labor environments by establishing minimum expectations for safety. Employees expect their place of employment to be reasonably safe, and managers have the responsibility to follow safety standards. The Occupational Safety and Health Administration (OSHA) oversees compliance and may inspect facilities for compliance. Any facility accidents must be properly documented, and this documentation is subject to review by OSHA. The Hazard Communication Standard says employees must be informed of chemical hazards present in the workplace. For each chemical, a material safety data sheet (MSDS) must be available that details the chemical hazards. Employees are also entitled to be made aware of any blood-borne pathogens to which they may be exposed while on the job.

FIRE SAFETY

The type of fire extinguisher used will depend upon the type of fire present.

- Water and foam extinguishers are used for Class A fires (combustible materials such as paper).
- Carbon dioxide extinguishers are used for Class B and C fires (flammable liquids and greases).
- Dry chemical extinguishers are used for Class A, B, and C fires (some effective for only Class B and C).
- Wet chemical extinguishers are Class K extinguishers designed for use in commercial kitchens.
- Clean agent (halon) extinguishers are used on Class B and C fires.
- Dry powder extinguishers are used for metal fires.

ACCIDENT PREVENTION

A food service safety program should consider engineering, education, and enforcement. The building and workspace should be engineered in a way that is safe, and likewise equipment should be properly installed and safe for use. Equipment should be maintained and replaced as needed. Workspace design should include equipment placement and good traffic flow. Education involves making safety procedures a priority for the staff. Safety policies and procedures must be discussed not only at job orientation but with ongoing training. Proper record keeping of accidents or injuries is also an aspect of education. All injuries and accidents need to be reported by employees and documented thoroughly. Finally, enforcement must be used to ensure compliance. The food service manager must assess whether safety protocols in place are working and take corrective action as needed. Although not all accidents are preventable, an accident-free workplace should be the goal.

PROPER DOCUMENTATION FOR WORKPLACE ACCIDENTS

According to the Occupational Safety and Health Administration, all workplace accidents or potential, near accidents are to be recorded. Employees should complete an accident form, and the form should be submitted to his/her supervisor. The purpose of recording is to have a document for corrective action and for reference. Details including where the accident took place, how it took place, and when it happened must be documented. Any equipment or tools that were being used at the time of the accident need to be described. Witnesses should be interviewed for a recount of the situation. The scenario and steps leading up to the accident must be recorded. It should be noted whether the accident was preventable and what steps may have prevented it. For example, an employee slips on the floor after it was mopped. It is determined there was no "wet floor" sign in place. The accident may have been prevented if proper signage had been placed. It should be determined whether a failure to follow procedures or a lack of proper safety procedures contributed to the accident. The injured body parts involved and whether medical attention was sought should be noted. The supervisor will review the employee form and complete a supervisor's form, followed by an investigation report. After a thorough investigation, corrective measures should be taken and documented.

Equipment and Facility Planning

Facility Layout

Equipment and Layout Planning

Menu

Equipment represents a major investment, and choices must be made wisely. The menu will drive the type of equipment needed for the operation, but costs, budget, facility size, and other factors will need to be considered before purchasing. Equipment will be based upon the types of foods being prepared, the restaurant setting, and the number of patrons served. An upscale restaurant with fresh meats and produce will have different equipment needs than a restaurant that uses many frozen and pre-prepared foods. Fresh meat and produce must have ample refrigerated storage space, and pre-prepared frozen foods require adequate freezer storage. Equipment used to prepare the foods will need to be considered. Gas ranges and griddle tops may be used to prepare meats, steaks, and sautéed vegetables for an upscale restaurant. Large and multiple ovens may be needed for reheating in a restaurant that uses pre-prepared foods. Pasta cookers may be useful for Italian-themed restaurants that prepare many pasta dishes. Meat slicers and bread ovens will be needed for sandwich shops, and deep fryers are common in fast-food restaurant serving fries.

Flow of Food

The facility layout and design will dictate the safety, efficiency, and effectiveness of an operation. A poor layout or design can be costly and have reoccurring adverse effects on the business. The kitchen design should reflect the anticipated workflow and incorporate the necessary equipment needed to carry out operations. Because equipment tends to be large, poor planning and building design may provide little room for error if large equipment is not accounted for in the planning phase. Workstations and equipment placement can affect work flow, which directly impacts efficiency. Once in place, rearranging large equipment may not be a feasible option. The kitchen layout and design will depend upon the service system used. A conventional system will have different needs than a commissary system. In a conventional operation, food is prepared and served on site. There will need to be a kitchen and a separate dining area in the facility. A commissary system will prepare mass quantities in one location and then transport the food to other locations. This may require a larger kitchen and more storage.

Safety and Sanitation

Considerations During Facility Design - Facilities should be designed with safety and sanitation in mind. Walls should be constructed of materials that are easily cleaned, and floors should be easy to clean and slip resistant for safety. Clay tiles are commonly used and generally considered the best option in high-traffic areas such as the kitchen. Proper ventilation is another consideration because it helps control humidity, which is an important criterion for proper food storage. Ample workspace is another important factor in design because it aids in workflow and efficiency. Aisles that need to accommodate more than one worker should be approximately 48 inches wide, and primary aisles should be at least 60 inches in width. When considering equipment purchases, ease of cleaning should be a factor in decision-making. Some equipment needs to be completely disassembled, whereas others may require partial disassembly to clean. Clean-in-place equipment is the easiest and requires no disassembly. Proper care and cleaning of equipment is essential in food safety, microbial control, and worker safety. The National Sanitation Foundation (NSF) is an independent organization that tests and certifies food service equipment. Equipment choices that meet NSF standards should be considered because equipment design, sanitation, and performance are evaluated when testing.

Dishwashing - Dishwashing may take place manually in a three-compartment sink or by using dishwashing machines. A three-compartment sink uses three compartments: one compartment to clean, one to rinse, and one to sanitize. If using a three-compartment sink, items must be sanitized by submersion using a chemical solution for one minute in 75°F water or submerged for 30 seconds in 170°F water. Mechanical dishwashers are used to easily and effectively clean dishes. Types of dishwashers include rack (items are placed on racks), conveyor belt (belt moves continuously through machine), and low-energy machines that use chemicals to sanitize instead of higher heat. Rack dishwashers are especially good for plates and glasses. The conveyor belt works best for smaller items such as silverware or other utensils.

Privacy and Accessibility

As with any place of business, privacy and accessibility are concerns. The facility should be accessible to patrons and workers but should be protected from those wishing to do harm. Safety and accessibility issues should ideally be addressed during the facility planning phase. The loading dock should be convenient for large trucks to enter. Placement of doors and entrances should be strategic and convenient. Limited access scanners can be placed near doors for added security to prevent unauthorized personnel. Storage areas should be conveniently located near the dock and kitchen areas but should also have safety measures such as locks and keypads to discourage unauthorized access. Because of the threat of bioterrorism or anyone wishing to do harm, access to work areas, food storage areas, and employee work rooms should be limited to authorized employees and necessary visitors only.

Codes and Standards

Impact on Facility Design/Build - During the planning phase, the planning team should understand local, state, and federal laws that impact the facility design, purpose, and location. Laws may vary by state and locality, but proper licensing and permits must be obtained. Building codes must be adhered to for safety purposes, and zoning laws will need to be explored before a site is chosen. Building permits must be issued, and inspections (electrical, plumbing, etc.) will need to be performed throughout the building process to ensure safety and code compliance. For food service operations, a health inspector will conduct an assessment of operations to ensure safety. Although the exact inspection criteria will vary by location, a critical aspect of the health inspection is food safety.

Impact of the ADA - Like other businesses, food service operations must adhere to the Americans with Disabilities Act (ADA). This law is meant to protect those with disabilities, such as individuals who are wheelchair bound. Because it is more difficult to get around in a wheelchair, accommodations should be made in the workplace and in the dining area to facilitate movement. Ramps will need to be installed to provide an alternative to stairs. Doors must be wide enough to accommodate a wheelchair, and aisles should be at least 3 feet wide. Dining table and chair placement needs to be considered to allow wheelchair movement. For the food service worker, shelves should be low enough to be accessible, and the workspace should be wide enough to allow for easy movement in the wheelchair. Restrooms must be designed to allow for wheelchair access and movement, and sinks/soap dispensers should be lower than standard height.

Planning Team

Composition and Roles/Responsibilities

Roles of the Planning Team in Facility Development - The assembled planning team will be instrumental in overseeing the facility's projects. The team may include the facility owner, food service manager, architects, designers, builders, contractors, business managers, and engineers. A written prospectus will guide the team throughout the process by providing a planning tool that details all aspects of the facility. The prospectus should explain the type of operation, the budget, location, equipment needs, layout considerations, safety objectives, and additional facts pertaining to the operation. Each team member will contribute to the plan using his/her area of expertise as a guide. For example, the architect may design the facility and recommend materials, whereas the engineer may focus on the safety aspects of the building's design. The builder or contractor will coordinate disciplines such as electricians and plumbers. The business manager and owner will be concerned with staying on budget and the timeliness of the project. The food service manager will likely be involved in many different aspects of the plan.

LEED Certification - Resource conservation has become a focus among many businesses and consumers. Building design and use can be organized with sustainability in mind—this has come to be known as green design. Green buildings can earn a Leadership in Energy and Environmental Design (LEED) Certification, and this is achieved by following certain standards aimed at sustainability and conservation. Conversation of resources has a positive impact on the environment by reducing the needs for fossil fuels, conserving water, and freeing up landfill space. In addition, meeting LEED standards can save the facility money by reducing electricity and water costs. Tax incentives may also be available to encourage a green design. Going green is not only socially responsible, but it is also good business. Responsible and sustainable business practices may result in greater customer loyalty and cost savings. Green practices take many forms, including using insulation to better maintain the climate in the facility. Solar panels may be installed to reduce the need for electricity. Equipment purchases can include designs that are more efficient and use less energy.

Equipment Specifications and Selection

Refrigerators are a major aspect and a major expense in a food service operation. Adequate refrigeration is essential, and the menu and type of operation will dictate refrigeration needs. Refrigeration needs should be decided during the planning phase of the operation. Built-in refrigerators are large, so placement and space are important considerations early in the planning phase. Depending on the operation and system used, a kitchen may require significant refrigerated space or may rely more on freezer space. An operation that prepares mostly fresh meats and vegetables will require more refrigeration than an operation that purchases frozen foods and reheats. Other considerations when purchasing include capacity, durability, and construction. Stainless steel is often used in food service equipment because it wears well and is easy to clean. When purchasing stainless steel appliances, metal gauge or thickness should be considered. Lower gauges indicate a stronger metal. Refrigeration systems should provide enough room to meet the storage needs of the operation and should be easy to clean to maintain food safety.

Sustainability

Conserving Resources

Food service operations can be major consumers of resources. Heating, cooling, and ventilation are big sources of resource drain on a building. Energy-efficient heating and cooling units can help conserve energy, and effective temperature control measures by personnel can further reduce consumption. Lighting use is another area in which conservation efforts may be focused. Buildings may be designed with windows and skylights to utilize natural night, and lights may be turned off or dimmed when not in use. Equipment design contributes to energy use, and how equipment is operated by staff also contributes to energy drain. Dishwashers that are run at less than full capacity waste water and electricity. Preheating equipment too soon is a drain on electricity and gas resources. Equipment should also be periodically inspected and kept in good working order to be most efficient. Conservation is a team effort; it starts in the design and planning phase and continues daily when the facility is fully operational.

Food and Water

Sustainability extends to food purchasing practices. Buying from suppliers that use sustainable practices is an important step in protecting the environment. For example, purchasing farm-raised salmon rather than wild-caught salmon is a practice that addresses overfishing and helps protect our ocean's ecosystems. Consider using vendors that purchase from small farms that grow sustainable crops by reducing or eliminating pesticide use and practice crop rotation.

Reducing water use in the operation is another step that can be taken to practice conservation. Efforts to reduce water waste should be explored because food service operations use a tremendous amount of water in daily operations for cooking and cleaning. Practices such as turning the water completely off and using toilets that conserve water are simple water-saving measures. Purchasing equipment that is energy efficient by means of recycling water is another way to conserve.

Non-Food

Supplies

Supplies used in daily food service operations may contribute heavily to environmental waste. Many operations utilize reusable plates, cups, and utensils, but others use disposable products to serve customers. Hospitals may use insulated foam containers to keep food warm for transport to the patient's room. Fast-food operations use a combination of foam, paper, and foil products to wrap and serve food and drink products. Unfortunately, many of these products used to hold and wrap food cannot be recycled after they are used. The exclusive use of paper, foam, and plastic contributes significantly to landfill waste, and this has a negative impact on the environment. An operation may go through hundreds or thousands of plastic, paper, and foam pieces on a daily basis. Common in food service organizations are supply packaging such as aluminum cans, glass containers, and cardboard from deliveries. These items can and should be recycled. Recycling these products is a responsible measure to help conserve natural resources and reduce landfill waste.

Waste Management

Storage and Disposal

Integrated solid waste management is a comprehensive approach using multiple avenues to practice waste management. No single approach can bring about the change needed, but managing waste through various practices can produce significant results for the environment. Landfills are not endless, so there is an urgent need to reduce the amount and size of trash. To help accomplish this, machines such as cardboard crushers, garbage disposals, and trash crushers can reduce the volume of trash going into the landfill. Recycling has multiple benefits, including conserving natural resources and reducing energy costs. To further reduce the amount of trash going into landfills, a recycling program should be undertaken by food service operations. Items such as aluminum, glass, plastic, paper, and foams can be recycled rather than thrown into the garbage. Rather than disposing of cooking oil, it can be sold and recycled into a usable biofuel. Yet another avenue to limit landfill trash is by composting unusable food waste. If excess food from production is usable, it may be used to make stocks or may be served the next day as a special menu offering. Composting is an alternative to throwing food scraps into the trash and is good for the soil and air. Incinerators may be used to burn waste, which limits the volume of materials placed in landfills.

Practice Test

1. What is the stored form of glucose?

a. Glycogen
b. Sucrose
c. Myoglobin
d. Monosaccharide

2. Which of the following is the minimum for wet diapers and stools expected daily for a properly fed breastfed infant?

a. 4 wet and 2 stools
b. 5 wet and 3 stools
c. 8 wet and 4 stools
d. 10 wet and 7 stools

3. Registered dietitians must adhere to which of the following to avoid losing their credentials?

a. Code of Ethics
b. Ethics and Morality Clause
c. Standards of Professional Conduct
d. Performance Standards

4. Which of the following is the appropriate first step in dealing with a food recall at your foodservice organization?

a. Communicating within the organization
b. Determining if food was served to the public
c. Communicating with the public
d. Providing a press release

5. How does Crohn's disease differ from Ulcerative Colitis?

a. Crohn's disease involves inflammation only in the large intestine
b. Ulcerative Colitis involves inflammation only in the large intestine
c. Weight loss is common with Crohn's disease but not with Ulcerative Colitis
d. Absorption is affected in Ulcerative Colitis but not in Crohn's disease

6. What type of sugar is created from the hydrolysis of sucrose?

a. Granulated table sugar
b. Raw Sugar
c. Invert Sugar
d. Corn Sugar

7. You have a 23-year-old female patient with a BMI of 16 along and reported recent weight loss. She appears very well educated and focused on nutrition; she also exercises intensely. Upon physical examination you notice the patient appears thin with lanugo hair on the skin. What do you suspect?

a. Anorexia Nervosa
b. Bulimia Nervosa
c. Type 1 diabetes
d. The patient is thin because of the intense exercise

8. What process is necessary to ensure the safety of milk?

a. Homogenization
b. Freezing
c. Irradiation
d. Pasteurization

9. There were complaints from customers about a cashier in the cafeteria. The cashier did not have a pleasant demeanor when dealing with customers. The cashier most likely lacked which of the following important skills?

a. Technical skills
b. Human skills
c. Leadership skills
d. Decision making skills

10. What type of food additive might a food manufacturer use to prevent a lumpy texture?

a. Stabilizer
b. Humectant
c. Salt
d. Leavening agent

11. The phrase "Calcium helps build strong bones" is an example of what type of label claim?

a. Health claim
b. Nutrient content claim
c. Structure/function claim
d. Cause/effect claim

12. You note from the labs that your patient has an eGFR of 14 mL per minute. What does this lab indicate?

a. Impaired kidney function
b. Normal kidney function
c. Chronic kidney failure
d. The patient is on dialysis

13. Which of the following individuals is most likely to have iron deficiency anemia?

a. An endurance athlete
b. Someone with congestive heart failure
c. Someone with irritable bowel syndrome
d. Someone with Celiac Disease

14. Which of the following is NOT the name of a specific test used to conduct sensory evaluations of food.

a. Duo-trio test
b. Hedonic scale
c. Descriptive testing
d. Texture scaling test

15. Consider a lunch line where customers go through the line and are served what is available rather than placing an order or specifying preferences. What type of menu is used in this establishment?

a. No-choice menu
b. Limited-choice menu
c. Single-use menu
d. Static menu

16. What is a potential advantage of genetically engineered foods?

a. Foods are proven safe
b. Foods are more natural
c. Foods may be more disease resistant
d. Foods are not FDA-regulated

17. Calculate the employee turnover ratio given a staff of 52 employees when 18 leave the organization.

a. 34.6 %
b. 28.8%
c. 25.2 %
d. 18%

18. What mineral works in conjunction with calcium to help build strong bones?

a. Vitamin D
b. Magnesium
c. Iron
d. Sulfur

19. In general, during the first trimester of pregnancy, how many more calories per day does a woman need?

a. 185 kcals per day
b. 340 kcals per day
c. 452 kcals per day
d. no additional calories are needed during the first trimester

20. Which of the following represents the type of production system where food is prepared at one site and transported to another site for serving?

a. Conventional
b. Commissary
c. Ready prepared
d. Transferal

21. Which process is most affected in individuals with type 1 diabetes?

a. Glycogenesis
b. Glycolysis
c. Krebs Cycle
d. Lactic Acid Cycle

22. Which of the follow does NOT occur when oils are hydrogenated?

a. Melting point is increased
b. Fat becomes more saturated
c. Shelf life of the product is increased
d. More molecular cis formations are created

23. You have decided to purchase sliced vegetables rather than whole vegetables for your restaurant. Which of the following parameters will be most affected?

a. Labor time
b. Quality
c. Cook time
d. Nutrient value

24. As a dietitian, you discover that your patient is having trouble meeting the weight loss goals set during your last counseling session. What should you do?

a. Reinforce the goals
b. Consider altering the goals
c. Re-educate the patient
d. Discharge the patient

25. Your department is working on the annual budget. You use last year's budget as a basis for the coming year. This type of budgeting is an example of which of the following?

a. Incremental budgeting
b. Performance budgeting
c. Zero-based budgeting
d. Historical budgeting

26. Motivational counseling might be appropriate for which of the following clients:

a. Someone who has a high level of education
b. Someone who wants to change
c. Someone who is a newly-diagnosed diabetic
d. Someone who is in denial about their diagnosis

27. As the food service director you notice productivity has been decreasing over the last 6 months. Which of the following actions would you first consider?

a. Hire more employees
b. Invest in new equipment
c. Evaluate the department training program
d. Look for ways to automate more processes

28. As a dietitian, what type of client might most benefit from a telehealth option?

a. A client with limited financial resources
b. A client who lives in a rural area
c. A client who lives in the city
d. A client who does not want to drive to the appointment

29. In which job is a smaller span of control appropriate?

a. Cook prep
b. Dishwashing
c. Nursing
d. Housekeeping

30. When should a product or program analysis be conducted?

a. Before product or program introduction
b. During program or product sales
c. Throughout the product or program lifecycle
d. After the product or program has ended

31. You are counseling a pregnant patient regarding weight gain during pregnancy. The pre-pregnancy BMI of your patient was 33.5. How much weight gain do you recommend for this patient?

a. 11-20 lbs.
b. 15-25 lbs.
c. 25-35 lbs.
d. 28-40 lbs.

32. During which of the follow steps of the Nutrition Care Process do you compare nutrition indicators against a comparative standard?

a. Assessment
b. Diagnosis
c. Intervention
d. Monitoring and Evaluation

33. Which of the following practices in most important in managing a diverse workforce?

a. Establishing rules
b. Having employee meetings
c. Practicing democratic leadership
d. Having an open dialogue

34. Your patient is 26 months of age. Which set of the following anthropometric measurements are important for this age?

a. Height and weight
b. Length and weight
c. Height, weight, and muscle mass
d. Height, weight, and head circumference

35. For the Family Medical Leave Act to be effective, an employee must have worked at the organization for which of the following lengths of time?

a. 6 months
b. 12 months
c. 8 months
d. 24 months

36. Which of the following foods would be most likely to inhibit the absorption of the thyroid medication, Synthroid?

a. White rice
b. Brussels sprouts
c. Peeled apples
d. Grapes

37. Which of the following could be considered the most important step in emergency management?

a. Response
b. Preparation
c. Coordination
d. Documentation

38. Which of the following foods is the best source of dietary vitamin E?

a. Nuts
b. Brown rice
c. Cheese
d. Chicken

39. Your patient has poorly controlled type 2 diabetes. In the past, this patient expressed no desire to change her eating habits. During your latest consult, she mentioned that she is now thinking about making dietary changes to better control her diabetes. At what behavior change stage is your patient?

a. Precontemplation
b. Contemplation
c. Determination
d. Action

40. Select the type of health surveillance that uses interviews and physical exams to ascertain information.

a. NHANES
b. BRFSS
c. YRBSS
d. CDCES

41. During a follow-up session with your client whom you are seeing for weight loss counseling, you weigh the client and determine that he has lost 7.5 lbs. since the last session. The client has achieved the set weight loss goal. This is an example of which of the following?

a. Nutrition Assessment
b. Nutrition Diagnosis
c. Nutrition Intervention
d. Monitoring and Evaluation

42. You check the stockroom and notice there are only 10 cans of corn remaining. You are required to maintain a stock of at least 12, so you must immediately order more. This minimum level is referred to as which of the following?

a. Minimum level
b. Cut off level
c. Stock level
d. Par level

43. According to the FDA Food Code, hot foods that will be stored should be cooled to 70 °F within how many hours?

a. 1 hour
b. 2 hours
c. 3 hours
d. 4 hours

44. Cuts of meat with a lot of collagen are best prepared using what type of cooking method?

a. Grilling
b. Frying
c. Stewing
d. Baking

45. Which of the following criteria most likely indicates Failure to Thrive (FTT) in an 18-month-old child?

a. Weight loss of 1-2 pounds
b. Weight falls from the 50th percentile to below the 10th percentile on the growth chart
c. The weight for length plots between the 5th and 10th percentile
d. Weight is at the 10th percentile for length/height

46. Which of the following is an example of protein coagulation?

a. Cooking a scrambled egg
b. Baking an apple pie
c. Cooking refried beans
d. Sautéing an onion

47. How is Celiac Disease definitively diagnosed?

a. Symptom investigation
b. Excluding gluten-containing foods from the diet
c. Intestinal biopsy
d. Blood laboratory test

48. Which of the following is NOT a function of management?

a. Planning
b. Organizing
c. Directing
d. Delegating

49. Which of the following factors will most affect the REE?

a. Fever
b. Moderate physical activity
c. Major surgery
d. Major burns

50. Which of the following foods may interfere with dietary iron absorption?

a. Whole grain pasta
b. Oranges
c. Fruit juice
d. White rice

51. An 81-year-old patient has been hospitalized following a stroke. The patient is progressing well, but you noticed him pocketing foods at mealtime. What course of action would you recommend?

a. None
b. Recommend a speech consult
c. Provide thickened liquids
d. Initiate a mechanically soft diet

52. Which of the following would NOT be permitted with a Kosher diet?

a. Beef
b. Salmon
c. Chicken
d. Shrimp

53. An egg with a normal-appearing shell, a firm yolk, and some thinning of the white is what grade of egg?

a. Grade AA
b. Grade A
c. Grade B
d. Grade AB

54. A patient has an LDL cholesterol of 159mg/dL and an HDL cholesterol of 39 mg/dL. Which of the following dietary interventions would you most recommend?

a. Limit saturated fat intake and increase fiber intake
b. Eliminate trans fats and increase protein intake
c. Initiate a weight loss program
d. Limit simple sugar intake

55. You have a supervisor who is very strict and dictatorial. He or she most likely believes in which of the following behavioral theories:

a. Theory W
b. Theory X
c. Theory Y
d. Theory Z

56. What type of insulin injection is typically given prior to meals and works quickly to help control blood glucose levels?

a. Bolus
b. Short-acting
c. Intermediate-acting
d. Long-acting

57. Which of the following food items would you discourage if the patient is following a low oxalate diet due to frequent kidney stone formation?

a. Wine
b. Milk
c. Grits
d. Beef

58. Which of the following nutrients will be most affected (destroyed or reduced) by cooking?

a. Vitamin B_6
b. Calcium
c. Magnesium
d. Vitamin C

59. Your 72-year-old male patient had a recent lab result suggesting vitamin B_{12} deficiency. Which of the following is the appropriate initial recommendation from the dietitian?

a. You recommend a vitamin B_{12} supplement
b. You recommend foods high in vitamin B_{12}
c. You refer the patient to his or her physician for follow-up
d. You recommend a daily multivitamin

60. Which of the following interventions may be appropriate for a patient with COPD?

a. Increase sodium intake
b. Decrease fat intake
c. Reduce carbohydrates intake
d. Increase overall caloric intake

61. Medicare Part B covers which of the following?

a. Hospital services
b. Professional services
c. Prescription drugs
d. Vision services

62. A clinical dietitian is considering expanding his or her clinical responsibilities in the hospital. Which of the following should first be considered?

a. Standards of Practice
b. Clinical Standards
c. Scope of Practice
d. Standards of Professional Performance

63. From the following choices, when should parenteral nutrition be considered?

a. After there has been insufficient intake for 7-14 days
b. When enteral nutrition is not successful
c. When the patient is being discharged for home care
d. After any type of bowel surgery

64. As a food service manager you order the needed items from various vendors based on their stated prices. This is an example of which of the following?

a. Competitive bidding
b. Open market bidding
c. No bidding
d. Flexible bidding

65. Regression analysis is used in what type of research?

a. Survey Research
b. Qualitative Research
c. Descriptive Research
d. Analytical Research

66. Which of the following is considered evidence for the presence of metabolic syndrome?

a. Rapid weight gain over a 1-year period accompanied by hypertension
b. Presence of diabetes and hypertension
c. Presence of diabetes, hypertension, and a BMI of 36
d. Presence of dyslipidemia and a BMI of 36

67. In addition to nutrition intervention, how are pressure ulcers best managed?

a. With repositioning and proper wound care dressings
b. With increased mobility
c. Through physical therapy
d. With proper bed positioning

68. Which of the following is not a key aspect of a food service safety program?

a. Engineering
b. Education
c. Enforcement
d. Environmental

69. Which of the following is the recommended time period for breastfeeding?

a. 0-3 months
b. 0-6 months
c. 12 months
d. 18 months

70. What gas can hasten the ripening process in some fruits (such as apples)?

a. Ethylene
b. Mylene
c. Phosphorylase
d. Methane

71. Using a standard enteral formula, your patient requires 2,000 kcals/day. Calculate bolus feeding amounts for 5 feedings daily.

a. 300 mL
b. 400 mL
c. 450 mL
d. 500 mL

72. What type of tube feeding would you recommend for a patient who needs some flexibility in feeding, but cannot tolerate large volumes in one sitting?

a. Bolus feeding
b. Continuous feeding
c. Intermittent feeding
d. Optional feeding

73. Which food ingredients do NOT need prior approval before including in foods?

a. Ingredients on the GRAS list
b. Color additives
c. New ingredient to market
d. Ingredients from an established food manufacturer

74. What nutrition program uses nutritional risk as a criterion for receiving services?

a. SNAP
b. Congregate Meals Program
c. Child and Adult Care Food Program
d. WIC

75. Which of the following groups has the highest BMR per body weight?

a. Infants
b. Children
c. Adolescents
d. Adults

76. Which of the following foods would you recommend for someone with PKU?

a. Milk
b. Hamburger patties
c. Nuts
d. Apples

77. A rural area with no grocery store within a 30-minute drive is known as which of the following?

a. Food desert
b. Food deprived area
c. Food challenged location
d. Food suburb

78. Which agency coordinates the national surveillance programs?

a. FDA
b. CDC
c. USDA
d. BRFSS

79. Energy needs are typically greatest during which part of infancy?

a. 0-3 months
b. 4-6 months
c. 7-12 months
d. Energy needs are not age dependent

80. A dietary supplement sold on TV claims to help you lose weight without exercise or calorie control. This is likely an example of which of the following?

a. Health fraud
b. Health fad
c. Health claim
d. Health promise

81. Approximately how many grams of carbohydrates would you find in a meal consisting of half a bagel, half a cup of orange juice and three-quarters of a cup of nonfat plain yogurt?

a. 30 g
b. 45 g
c. 60 g
d. 65 g

82. Which of the following is considered a risk factor for heart disease?

a. Having HDL cholesterol less than 40 mg/dL
b. Having HDL cholesterol greater than 40 mg/dL
c. Being a male over 40 years of age
d. Being a female over 45 years of age

83. Your organization is planning to build a new hospital wellness wing starting in 3 years. This example illustrates which type of planning?

a. Short term planning
b. Long-range planning
c. Operational planning
d. Structure planning

84. Which of the following is an example of a departmental procedure?

a. Proper work attire
b. Specifications for how to properly document client information
c. Work day schedules
d. Behavior expectations

85. Your 42-year-old male patient has a Hgb of 12 with no significant medical history. Which of the following foods would you recommend this patient eat to address the hemoglobin?

a. Garden salad with cheese
b. Rice and beans
c. Toast with fruit
d. Chicken with broccoli

86. Which of the following is an example of a staff role?

a. Accountant
b. Customer service representative
c. Nurse
d. Line server

87. You have just completed a 6-week educational series on cardiovascular health for your cardiac rehabilitation patients. What would you use to assess the program's success?

a. Periodic Evaluation
b. Peer Evaluation
c. Summative Evaluation
d. Formative Evaluation

88. Which of the following management styles would you choose to help a new employee who is very motivated but lacks experience?

a. Coaching
b. Directive
c. Supportive
d. Delegating

89. Which of the following tends to be the most accurate and comprehensive method of obtaining dietary intake for a patient?

a. 24-hour recall
b. Food frequency questionnaire
c. Food diary
d. Food survey

90. What process or processes can help preserve the bright green color in foods such as green beans?

a. Chlorophyll
b. Blanching and freezing
c. Heating
d. Ripening

91. The line item *Sales* would be included in which of the following types of budgets?

a. Capital budget
b. Operating budget
c. Essential budget
d. Expenditure budget

92. You just completed a training for newly-diagnosed diabetes patients. After the training, you discovered some of the participants have very low literacy and did not understand some of your educational materials. What should you have done to avoid this situation?

a. Asked the patients if they could read or understand the materials
b. Conducted a needs assessment
c. Involved family members in the training
d. Provided fewer handouts

93. On which financial statement would you find the organization's assets listed?

a. Income statement
b. Balance sheet
c. Statement of Cash Flows
d. Statement of Retained Earnings

94. Healthcare facilities such as hospitals often strive to achieve which of the following certifications?

a. NCQA
b. JCAHO
c. HHS
d. AHA

95. What type of fish should pregnant women avoid eating?

a. Shrimp
b. Salmon
c. Swordfish
d. Tilapia

96. Opportunity costs are defined as which of the following?

a. How much a new opportunity will cost in dollars
b. The cost of capital
c. The loss of potential benefit when pursuing one option
d. Benefits that a new opportunity will provide

97. You received a referral because the hospital screening tool indicated a 78-year-old male is malnourished. He was hospitalized for complications resulting from influenza. Upon assessment, you determine the patient has a BMI of 18 with recent weight loss. The patient has no history of cardiovascular disease or diabetes. He lives alone and is able to purchase and prepare foods, but he says his appetite is poor and food is lacking in taste. What first course of intervention might you recommend for this patient?

a. DASH diet
b. Bolus feedings combined with oral intake
c. Normal diet with high-calorie supplements
d. Liberalized diet

98. Tube feeding is initiated in a severely malnourished patient. You should carefully monitor for which of the following:

a. Weight loss
b. Fluid loss
c. Refeeding Syndrome
d. Overfeeding Syndrome

99. The patient is hospitalized post cholecystectomy. What type of diet would you first recommend post-surgery?

a. Nothing by mouth
b. High-fat diet
c. Low-fat diet
d. Regular diet

100. Which is the following is the first step a dietitian should take to address the needs of a burn patient?

a. Replace fluids
b. Start enteral nutrition
c. Start parenteral nutrition
d. Begin supplemental zinc sulfate

101. You are a clinical manager for the food and nutrition department at your local hospital. One of your clinical dietitians is being called away for active-duty military service, but she plans to return after 6 months. Upon her return from service, which of the following actions would you take?

a. Reemploy her in the same or equivalent position
b. Reemploy her if there is an opening
c. Assist the dietitian in finding a job at another hospital
d. Provide severance pay and a letter of recommendation

102. Your 20-year-old male patient has a BMI of 25.9. Which BMI classification is this patient in?

a. Underweight
b. Normal weight
c. Overweight
d. Obese

103. You are managing a large foodservice operation and you need to be profitable to continue in business. Your net income is $50,000, your net sales are $90,000, and your cost of goods sold is $24,000. Calculate the profit margin.

a. 48%
b. 55%
c. 180%
d. 375%

104. You, the clinical dietitian, stop in to follow up with your 5th floor patient. The patient is feeling much better, but he complains of being hungry now that his appetite is returning. You note the patient is on a reduced sodium diet, but there are no other restrictions. Rather than ordering a food supplement or snack for the patient, you walk to the kitchen, pick up the food, and deliver it to the patient. This scenario is best described as of which of the following?

a. Customer service
b. Team work
c. Outside the scope of practice
d. Within the standards of care

105. A patient is diagnosed with galactosemia and referred to the dietitian. Which of the following foods would you recommend eliminating from the diet based on the diagnosis?

a. Yogurt
b. Sugar
c. Fresh meat
d. Eggs

106. What monosaccharides join to form sucrose?

a. Glucose and maltose
b. Fructose and galactose
c. Fructose and lactose
d. Fructose and glucose

107. Your patient has ESRD and is on hemodialysis. Which of the following most likely reflects the appropriate amount of protein to be consumed by this patient?

a. 1.6 g/kg/day
b. 1.4 g/kg/day
c. 1.2 g/kg/day
d. 0.8 g/kg/day

108. You have an employee away on family medical leave. You need to hire someone to fill in for the employee while he is absent. This new hire is probably which of the following types of employees?

a. Probationary employee
b. Part-time employee
c. Short-term worker
d. Temporary worker

109. Your 83-year-old low-income female patient is being discharged from the hospital. She has limited transportation and no family. Which of the following services would be most appropriate for this patient?

a. USDA Commodity Supplemental Food Program
b. WIC Program
c. Senior Farmer's Market Nutrition Program
d. Supplemental Nutrition Assistance Program

110. When preparing a menu, which of the following is NOT a factor that would likely be considered?

a. Budget
b. Clientele
c. Food service equipment
d. Dining room ergonomics

111. Your patient is post-gastric bypass and experiencing dumping syndrome. Which of the following recommendations would you make?

a. Drink more fluids such as fruit juice
b. Chew more slowly
c. Add fluids, especially milk products
d. Provide protein foods

112. Your restaurant changes menus every spring, summer, fall, and winter. These menus are known as which of the following types of menus?

a. Seasonal
b. Yearly
c. Preferred
d. Evolving

113. When should you consider total parenteral nutrition?

a. When feeding is short term (3-4 days in duration)
b. When longer-term feeding is expected (over 7 days in duration)
c. After bowel surgery that requires nothing by mouth for 1 – 2 days
d. When the patient is reluctant to eat by mouth

114. Your hospital is adopting a new electronic medical record system. How would you best begin the training for the new system?

a. New employee orientation
b. Written instructions
c. In-Service
d. On-the-job training

115. Nutrition-related knowledge deficit is an example of which nutrition diagnosis domain?

a. Intake
b. Clinical
c. Behavioral-environmental
d. Educational

116. To destroy which of the following bacteria, vegetables must be canned at a temperature above 212 °F?

a. Clostridium botulinum
b. E. coli
c. Salmonella
d. Listeria

117. Which of the following is NOT a reason why a foodservice organization should follow standardized recipes?

a. Consistent product
b. Quality
c. Less time consuming
d. Cost control

118. Which of the following is an example of a food fad?

a. Mediterranean diet
b. Cardiac prudent diet
c. Low carbohydrate diet
d. DASH diet

119. For how long should one scrub hands when following proper handwashing procedures?

a. 60 seconds
b. 30 seconds
c. 20 seconds
d. 15 seconds

120. A patron is sick with diarrhea and cramping after eating a fresh salad at your restaurant 3 days ago. Which of the following food borne illnesses is most likely responsible for the symptoms?

a. Salmonella
b. E. coli
c. Trichinosis
d. Listeria

121. During which phase of the Nutrition Care Process does implementation take place?

a. Nutrition Assessment
b. Nutrition Diagnosis
c. Nutrition Intervention
d. Nutrition Monitoring and Evaluation

122. You notice that blood levels are becoming acidic in a patient on a ventilator. This condition is known as which of the following?

a. Respiratory Acidosis
b. Respiratory Alkalosis
c. Metabolic Acidosis
d. Metabolic Alkalosis

123. The act of trying to prevent bioterrorism that may occur through food supply contamination is known as which of the following?

a. Food safety
b. Supply safety
c. Food defense
d. Supply defense

124. Which of the following would NOT be found on a clear liquid diet.

a. Tea
b. Apple juice
c. Orange juice
d. Ice pops

125. A commissary food production system will require which of the following?

a. A large kitchen
b. A large dining area
c. Limited storage
d. Specialized equipment

Answer Key and Explanations

1. A: Glycogen is the stored form of glucose and is classified as a polysaccharide. Sucrose is a disaccharide sugar. Monosaccharides are a class of sugar, but not the stored form of glucose. Myoglobin is not a sugar.

2. B: Breastfed infants are expected to have at least 5 wet diapers and 3 stools per day. Monitoring the number of wet diapers and stools provides an indication of adequate intake. Typically, breastfed infants have more stools than formula-fed infants.

3. A: Like many professional organizations, the Academy of Nutrition and Dietetics has a Code of Ethics that must be followed by professionals within the organization.

4. A: Details of the recall need to first be communicated throughout the organization, including any satellite sites. Once everyone has the appropriate information, it can be determined whether any food was actually served to the public. If so, then the public should be notified if there is any danger.

5. B: Ulcerative Colitis involves inflammation of the large intestines; Crohn's disease may involve inflammation in any part of the digestive tract. In both, absorption is affected and weight loss is a concern.

6. C: Invert Sugar is created from the breakdown of sucrose in water to form a mixture of glucose and fructose; invert sugars are often used in syrups. Sucrose is used to form granulated table sugar. Neither raw sugar or corn sugar are formed from a combination of two or more sugars.

7. A: Anorexia Nervosa is a possibility. A BMI less than 18.5 indicates that the patient is underweight. The patient also appears very informed about food and exercises intently. These are often characteristics of someone with anorexia (when coupled with other factors). Finally, the patient has lanugo -- a fine body hair that often covers patients suffering from anorexia nervosa.

8. D: Pasteurization kills microbes by heating the milk to high temperatures. Homogenization is a part of milk processing, but it does not destroy pathogens; rather it prevents the fat from separating from the liquid.

9. B: The cashier probably lacks human skills, which are helpful when interacting and dealing with coworkers and customers. This employee may benefit from customer service training or placement in a role that does not directly interact with customers.

10. A: Stabilizers such as gelatin are used to prevent lumps and separation. Humectants, salts, and leavening agents are also food additives but their purposes are not to prevent a lumpy texture.

11. C: Structure function claims relate a nutrient to a bodily function. A health claim is different in that it indicates a relationship between a food and a medical condition.

12. C: Chronic kidney failure is indicated by an eGFR of less than 15 mL per minute. At this stage, dialysis or kidney transplantation are the only treatment options.

13. D: Celiac Disease can result in poor dietary absorption. Irritable bowel syndrome may cause discomfort when eating, but it does not automatically predispose someone to iron deficiency anemia, and nutrient absorption is not affected.

14. D: Texture scaling is not the name of a specific test used to conduct sensory evaluations. The other choices use a panel of judges to assess food qualities and characteristics.

15. A: A no-choice menu is being used because the patrons have no choice about what food will be plated for them. This type of menu is often used in school cafeterias.

16. C: Genetically modified foods can be engineered to resist disease. This has economic benefits because of a greater crop yield. The FDA **does** regulate genetically modified foods as they do other foods, but public concerns over safety remain. Although safety is not absolutely proven, there is evidence to suggest genetically modified foods are safe for consumption.

17. A: The calculation is as follows:

$$\frac{\text{Number of employees who left or were terminated}}{\text{total number of employees in department}} \times 100$$

$$\frac{18}{52} \times 100 = 34.6\%$$

18. B: Magnesium works with calcium in bone metabolism; magnesium is necessary for parathyroid hormone secretion. Vitamin D is important for strong bones, but it is a vitamin not a mineral.

19. D: Energy requirements do not increase during the first trimester of pregnancy. During the second trimester an estimated 340 kcals per day are needed, and during the third trimester a woman needs an additional 452 kcals per day.

20. B: Commissary production is where there is a central location for preparation, and the prepared foods are moved to different sites for serving. This setup is often used to avoid the cost of having multiple sites for food prep, thus commissary production can result in cost containment.

21. A: Glycogenesis is impacted the most because insulin, which stimulates glucokinase, is not readily available. Therefore, glucokinase levels are not sufficient; glucokinase is instrumental in the liver's metabolism of glucose.

22. D: All of the above occur except D, the creation of more cis formations. When oils are hydrogenated, more molecular trans formations are created, not molecular cis formations.

23. A: Labor time will change the most. Vegetables that are already sliced save the labor time which would have been spent slicing whole vegetables.

24. B: You should consider altering the goals since goals are not set in stone. You may need to reassess and discover why the patient his not meeting his or her goals. Perhaps the goals were too aggressive and you need to set more realistic goals.

25. A: Using last year's budget as a basis for the upcoming budget is an example of incremental budgeting. An incremental budget is based on historical data and is used when few changes are expected from year to year.

26. B: Someone who wants to change would be a good candidate for motivational counseling. People who have the desire to make changes often need a motivator to help facilitate those changes. Someone who is newly-diagnosed or in denial about their diagnosis may not be ready for motivational counseling.

27. C: You should first consider the adequacy of the training program. A lack of proper training can have a negative impact on employee productivity.

28. B: A client who lives in a rural area with limited access to a dietitian or other healthcare provider is most likely to benefit from telehealth.

29. C: A smaller span of control is appropriate with nursing care because nursing professionals do many different tasks.

30. A: The analysis should occur before the product's release and before a program is introduced. Analysis prior to introduction helps improve the odds for success because it will identify barriers and facilitators for success.

31. A: The patient is classified as obese, so a lower weight gain range of 11-20 lbs. is recommended compared to individuals of underweight, normal, or overweight status.

32. A: Assessment is the phase where information on the patient is gathered. That information should be compared with the appropriate reference standard for comparison.

33. D: Maintaining an open dialogue is probably most important when managing a diverse workforce. Open dialogue can facilitate amicable, productive discussion.

34. D: Height, weight, and head circumference should be measured in children under 36 months of age. After 36 months of age, head circumference is no longer measured.

35. B: An employee who has worked for an organization for at least 12 months is eligible for family medical leave.

36. B: Brussels sprouts are very high in fiber. Fiber can inhibit the absorption of the thyroid medication, Synthroid.

37. B: Preparation is likely the most important step in emergency management. You must first prepare for the emergency. An appropriate response would be unlikely if there is not adequate emergency preparation.

38. A: Vitamin E is a fat-soluble vitamin which is abundant in nuts and oils. Although cheese may be high in fat, it is not a significant source of vitamin E. The other choices provide only a trace amount or insignificant amount of vitamin E.

39. B: Currently, this patient is in the Contemplation phase. The patient is contemplating or thinking about making a change. Previously, the patient was in the Precontemplation phase and not considering a change, but she has progressed since that time.

40. A: NHANES is a unique surveillance program in that information is gathered through interviews and physical exams. The other programs do not include a physical exam, and CDCES is not a surveillance program.

41. D: Monitoring and evaluation is the correct answer because you are comparing outcomes (lost 7.5 lbs.) to interventions (weight loss counseling).

42. D: Par level is the minimum amount allowed, in this case 12. When the stock falls below par level, more items must be ordered. This helps avoid shortages.

43. B: Food should be cooled to 70 °F within 2 hours. Time within the 'danger zone' where bacteria can grow needs to be limited to maintain food safety.

44. C: Stewing is the correct answer. Foods with a lot of collage benefit from a moist heat type of cooking such as stewing. Collagen is a tough connective tissue which needs time to break down during the cooking process. The slower cooking time and moisture help soften the tough tissue.

45. B: When the weight falls more than two growth channels, FTT should be suspected.

46. A: Cooking a scrambled egg is an example of protein coagulation. The liquid from the yolk and egg white turns solid in a process known as coagulation.

47. C: The only definitive way to diagnose Celiac disease is through an intestinal biopsy. This is often not performed because it is invasive and expensive. The presence of antibodies in the blood can suggest the presence of Celiac disease, but it is not definitive indicator.

48. D: Delegating may be used as a means of leading or directing, but it is not a main function of management.

49. D: Major burns will most affect Resting Energy Expenditure, which is a measure of metabolic rate. Burns have a tremendous effect on the body and cause a significant stress response.

50. A: Whole grain pasta is most likely to interfere with iron absorption because it is high in fiber content, and fiber can inhibit the absorption of iron. Vitamin C may aid the absorption of iron.

51. B: You suspect swallowing difficulty or dysphagia post-stroke. A speech consult should be recommended to assess if there is a swallowing problem. The diet order or recommendation should reflect the outcome of the speech therapy findings.

52. D: Shellfish, including shrimp, would not be permitted on a Kosher diet.

53. B: Grade A is typically what you see on the grocery store shelves. Grade AA is the highest quality while Grade B is lower quality and typically has more defects. Grade AB is not an egg grade.

54. A: Saturated fats should be limited to less than 7% of calories and fiber intake should be increased by eating whole grains, fruits, and vegetables.

55. B: This supervisor most likely subscribes to Theory X. Theory X asserts that most people do not want to work and are not motivated; hence the supervisor exercises strict control over employees in order to force them to work.

56. A: A bolus injection is generally given before meals. The dosage is based on the planned amount of carbohydrates consumed at the meal.

57. C: Grits are high in oxalate; the other choices are considered low-oxalate items.

58. D: Vitamin C is greatly affected by heat, so losses of this nutrient can be expected during the cooking process. The B vitamins are generally more heat-stable. Minerals are less affected by heat than vitamins.

59. C: You should refer the patient to his physician to discuss the appropriate treatment. In the elderly, vitamin B_{12} deficiency is often due to a lack of intrinsic factor. While a supplement containing B_{12} or foods high in B_{12} may be useful, the patient will likely need B_{12} injections if absorption is altered due to lack of intrinsic factor.

60. D: An increase in caloric intake may be necessary because the metabolic rate increases in individuals with COPD. Malnutrition is often a problem among this population. Sodium should generally be limited and healthy fats can be liberalized. Restricting carbohydrates may not be beneficial.

61. B: Medicare Part B covers professional services such as doctor visits and durable medical equipment.

62. C: Dietitians must be careful to operate within their scope of practice. According to the Academy, the scope of practice, "encompasses the range of roles, activities, and regulations within which nutrition and dietetics practitioners perform." The scope of practice takes into account many considerations including education, credentialing, and competence.

63. B: Parenteral nutrition should be considered after enteral nutrition is unsuccessful. Enteral nutrition should be the first choice following intake by mouth. Some types of bowel surgery may necessitate the need for parental nutrition, but this is not always the case.

64. B: This is known as open market bidding because you are not tied to one vendor. With competitive bidding one vendor is chosen to supply the food service needs.

65. D: Analytical research involves understanding and making predictions. Regression analysis is a method that attempts to show a correlation between variables.

66. C: Metabolic syndrome is considered when there are multiple symptoms (three or more) such as hyperglycemia, obesity or high waist circumference, hypertension, and dyslipidemia. The other answers include only two symptoms and choice 'A' includes a characteristic that does not meet the criteria of rapid weight gain.

67. A: Although a lack of mobility may contribute to pressure ulcers, the ulcer patient must be repositioned frequently and the wounds must be properly dressed in order to effectively treat the condition.

68. D: Environmental is not a key aspect of a food service safety program. The building should be engineered to promote safety, the staff should be educated, and the rules should be enforced to promote a safe environment.

69. C: The recommendation is for infants to be breastfed for the first 12 months of life, but any amount of breastfeeding is encouraged because of the numerous health benefits.

70. A: Fruits naturally produce ethylene gas, which speeds up the ripening process. Mylene is not a gas, and phosphorylase is an enzyme. Methane is a flammable gas that is a component of natural gas, which is often used for heating and cooking.

71. B: 2,000 kcals = 2,000 mL standard formula at 1 kcal/mL. $\frac{2{,}000 \text{ mL}}{5 \text{ feedings}} = 400\frac{\text{mL}}{\text{feeding}}$

72. C: Intermittent feeding would be appropriate because it is offered several times daily and is more flexible than continuous feeding. Bolus feeding would not be recommended because the patient is unable to tolerate large volumes.

73. A: Ingredients on the Generally Recognized as Safe (GRAS) list do not need prior approval before inclusion in foods. Safety is assumed for these ingredients given the number of years on the market without adverse effect coupled with scientific support.

74. D: The Special Supplemental Food Program for Women, Infants, and Children (WIC) is the only program that requires nutrition risk be established prior to receiving services.

75. A: Infants have the highest Basal Metabolic Rate based on their body weight. Infants grow very quickly and need a tremendous amount of energy.

76. D: Fruits are low in phenylalanine, which must be limited in patients with PKU. Milk and dairy products, meats, and nuts are higher in phenylalanine and should be avoided.

77. A: A food desert is an area without easy access to fresh fruits and vegetables. A food desert may be found in rural or more urban areas. In urban areas you might find stores that offer packaged or preserved food but lack healthy, fresh options. In rural areas there may be no food options.

78. B: The Centers for Disease Control (CDC) coordinate surveillance programs such as the Behavioral Risk Factor Surveillance System (BRFSS) and the Youth Risk Behavior Surveillance System (YRBSS).

79. A: During the first three months of life energy needs respective to weight are the greatest. Energy needs for this age span are calculated with the following equation:

$$EER\left(\frac{kcal}{day}\right) = (89 \times infant\ weight\ in\ kg - 100) + 175.$$

80. A: This scenario is an example of health fraud. This product is not supported by science and attempts to make a profit using misinformation.

81. B: Approximately 45 grams of carbohydrates will be included in this meal because each item contains about 15 grams of carbohydrates.

82. A: Low HDL cholesterol is considered a risk factor for heart disease. HDL cholesterol is often referred to as "good" cholesterol because it helps remove harmful cholesterol from the body.

83. B: This is an example of long-range planning. Long range planning looks into the future beyond a year.

84. B: Specifications for how to document client information is an example of a procedure. A procedure describes *how* something should be done; there are steps that must be followed for proper documentation. The other choices are examples of policies.

85. D: A hemoglobin level of 12 is considered low for a male. Chicken and broccoli would be the best recommendation. Chicken is a good source of dietary iron, while broccoli contains a significant amount of vitamin C. Vitamin C helps increase the absorption of iron.

86. A: An accountant is an example of a staff role; he or she does not have a direct impact on the customer.

87. C: A summative evaluation is given at the end of a period or series of programs. It helps to evaluate or summarize the entire program rather than just one class within the program. A formative evaluation might be used for only one class or counseling session so changes can be made moving forward.

88. B: You would likely choose a coaching style. The coaching style utilizes both support and direction; this is important for a new, inexperienced employee.

89. C: A food diary is generally more accurate than a 24-hour recall because it relies less on a person's memory. A food frequency questionnaire provides limited information in that it looks at how frequently a food is eaten; whereas a food diary should include all intake. A food survey is not considered a method of obtaining intake information for a specific patient.

90. B: Blanching vegetables prior to freezing can help maintain their coloring that results from the pigment chlorophyll. Heating generally causes a loss of color in chlorophyll-pigmented foods. Colors usually become brighter during the ripening process.

91. B: An operating budget includes line items such as sales and labor. A capital budget includes major expenses such as equipment and buildings.

92. B: If you had conducted the needs assessment prior to the education session, you could have assessed the needs and education level of your group. This would have allowed you to provide handouts aimed at a lower literacy level.

93. B: A balance sheet is frequently used by outside entities or persons for investment decisions. It details information such as assets, liability and owner's equity.

94. B: The Joint Commission on Accreditation of Healthcare Agencies (JCAHO) offers certification for healthcare facilities. While their accreditation is not a requirement, it is an industry standard for quality.

95. C: Swordfish should be avoided because it is higher in mercury.

96. C: Opportunity cost is what you give up when you pursue an alternate option. When you conduct a cost/benefit analysis, part of the analysis includes opportunity cost.

97. C: Because there is no mention of contraindication to oral feeding, a normal diet combined with high calorie supplements is likely the best course of initial action.

98. C: You should monitor for refeeding syndrome. This life-threatening scenario may occur when initiating feeding after prolonged periods of malnourishment. The patient should be followed closely and labs should be monitored especially for increases in phosphate, potassium, glucose, and magnesium.

99. C: Initially, the patient should be on a low-fat diet and progress as tolerated to a regular diet. The gallbladder stores and releases bile; bile is important in the metabolism of fats. With the removal of the gallbladder this process is disturbed, so following a low-fat diet is important. Eventually, the liver will compensate for the absence of the gallbladder.

100. A: Much fluid is lost in burn patients; the appropriate first step is to replace fluids. Enteral nutrition may be necessary if the patient is unable to initiate feedings by mouth. Supplemental zinc sulfate should be recommended, but these occur secondary to correcting fluid loss.

101. A: Under the Uniformed Services Employment and Reemployment Act, employees have the right to return to their previous position or an equivalent position if they remain qualified.

102. C: A BMI of 25-29 is considered overweight for male and female adults.

103. C: $Profit\ Margin\ = \frac{\text{Net Income}}{\text{Net Sales}}$

$$\frac{50{,}000}{90{,}000} = 0.55 = 55.5\%$$

This means your food service operation has 55.5% of your revenue remaining after direct costs (such as food) are paid. Net income already has cost of goods sold subtracted, so you do not need this number.

104. A: This is an example of good customer service. The dietitian could have ordered a food supplement or snack to be delivered at a later time by the food service staff. Instead, he or she went above and beyond to provide excellent service to the patient.

105. A: Yogurt should be avoided because it contains lactose (galactose is found in lactose). Individuals with galactosemia lack the necessary enzyme to metabolize galactose.

106. D: Fructose and glucose form sucrose when joined, which is commonly referred to as table sugar.

107. C: 1.2 g/kg/day is the protein intake typically suggested for patients receiving hemodialysis. The protein needs may be higher for patients receiving peritoneal dialysis.

108. D: Temporary workers are often hired on a short-term basis to fill in for someone who is absent or to supplement work for a particular period of time (for instance, to help fill the gaps during the busy season).

109. A: The USDA Commodity Supplemental Food Program would be appropriate because it delivers food to the home. This is important because the patient has limited means of transportation.

110. D: While dining room ergonomics are important when designing the space and for comfort, it is unlikely to be a factor you will consider when planning a menu.

111. D: Protein-containing foods such as chicken and beef are digested more slowly and should be emphasized. Fruit juice may make the dumping syndrome worse while lactose-containing products such as milk may be difficult to digest.

112. A: Menus that change based on the season are referred to as seasonal menus. Patrons often prefer different foods at different times of the year. A hot cup of soup is nice in the cold winter, but in the summer, someone may prefer something more refreshing. In addition, seasonal menus are good because it allows the food service operation to serve fresh foods that are in season.

113. B: Total parenteral nutrition is generally considered for longer term situations. PPN should be used for shorter durations if the patient is unable to tolerate intake by mouth or enteral feeding by tube.

114. C: An in-service or a series of in-service sessions should be scheduled to train employees on how to use the new medical record system. Written instructions may be helpful, but they should not be the only mode of training. The employees should be comfortable with the system prior to implementation; therefore, on the job training is not the optimal choice.

115. C: A knowledge deficit falls into the behavioral-environmental category of nutrition diagnoses. While a knowledge deficit might be related to a lack of education, Educational is not considered a nutrition diagnosis domain.

116. A: Vegetables, because they are lower in acid and prone to microbial growth, must be canned at very high temperatures to destroy the harmful bacterium, clostridium botulinum.

117. C: Following a standardized recipe may or may not be less time-consuming than the alternative. It is not a reason for using standardized recipes, but controlling costs and producing a high quality, consistent product are reasons.

118. C: A low-carbohydrate diet is an example of a food fad. The low-carbohydrate approach restricts carbohydrates unnecessarily and is not based on sound scientific principles.

119. C: Proper handwashing procedures recommend scrubbing for 20 seconds.

120. B: If the symptoms are from a food borne illness, the most likely culprit from our choices is E. coli. E. coli can be found in beef products as well as fresh fruits and vegetables.

121. C: During Nutrition Intervention the dietitian puts his/her plan into practice and implements the strategies.

122. A: Respiratory acidosis has likely resulted from inefficient breathing causing a build-up of carbon dioxide. Metabolic acidosis also results in a decreased pH, but metabolic acidosis is involved with kidney function.

123. C: Preventative measures and training to prevent bioterrorism as related to food, is known as food defense.

124. C: Orange juice would generally not be found on a clear liquid diet. A clear liquid diet can include fruit juices such as apple juice, but it excludes juices with pulp such as orange juice.

125. A: A commissary system will require a large kitchen. Large quantities of food are being prepared on-site and transported to satellite locations for serving.

Special Report: Normal Lab Values

<u>For Reference Purposes</u>

Hematologic

Bleeding Time (Template): Less than 10 minutes

Erythrocyte count: 4.2 -5.9 million/cu mm

Erythrocyte sedimentation rate (Westergren): Male- 0-15mm/hr; Female: 0-20mm/hr

Hematocrit, blood: Male- 42-50%; Female: 40-48%

Hemoglobin, blood: Male-13-16 g/dL; Female- 12-15 g/dL

Leukocyte count and differential

- Leukocyte count: 4000-11,000/ cu mm
- 50-70% segmented neutrophils
- 0-5% band forms
- 0-3 % eosinophils
- 0-1% basophils
- 30-45% lymphocytes
- 0-6% monocytes

Mean corpuscular volume: 86-98 fL

Prothrombin time, plasma: 11-13 seconds

Partial thromboplastin time (activated): 30-40 seconds

Platelet count: 150,000-300,000/ cu mm

Reticulocyte count: 0.5-1.5% of red cells

Whole Blood, Plasma, Serum Chemistries

Amylase, serum: 25-125 U/L

Arterial studies, blood (patient breathing room air)

- PO_2 : 75-100 mm Hg
- PCO_2 : 38-42 mm Hg
- Bicarbonate: 23-26 mEq/L
- pH: 7.38-7.44
- Oxygen saturation: 95% or greater

Bilirubin, serum

- Total: 0.3-1.0 mg/dL
- Direct: 0.1-0.3 mg/dL

Comprehensive metabolic panel:

- Bilirubin, serum (total): 0.3-1.0 mg/dL
- Calcium, serum: Male: 9.0-10.5 mg/dL; Female: 8.5-10.2 mg/dL
- Chloride, serum: 98-106 mEq/L
- Cholesterol, serum (total):
- Desirable: less than 200mg/dL
- Borderline-high: 200-239 mg/dL (may be high in the presence of coronary artery disease or other risk factors)
- High: greater than 239 mg/dL
- Creatine, serum: 0.7-1.5 mg/dL
- Glucose, plasma:
- Normal (fasting)- 70-115 mg/dL
- Borderline: 115-140 mg/dL
- Abnormal: greater than 140 mg/dL
- Phosphorus, serum: 3.0-4.5 mg/dL
- Proteins, serum:
- Pre-Albumin: 0.2-0.4 g/dL
- Albumin: 3.5-5.5 g/dL
- Urea nitrogen, blood (BUN): 8-20 mg/dL
- Uric acid, serum: 3.0 7.0 mg/dL

High-density lipoprotein: Low- less than 200 mg/dL

Low-density lipoprotein:

- Optimal: less than 100 mg/dL
- Near-optimal: 100-129 mg/dL
- Borderline-high: 130-159 mg/dL (may be high in the presence of coronary artery disease or other risk factors)
- High: 160-189 mg/dL
- Very high: 190 mg/dL and above

Electrolytes, serum:

- Sodium: 136-145 mEq/L
- Potassium: 3.5-5.0 mEq/L
- Chloride: 98-106 mEq/L
- Bicarbonate: 23-28 mEq/L

Follicle-stimulating hormone, serum:

- Male: 2-18 mIU/mL
- Female:
- 5-20 mIU/mL (follicular or luteal)
- 30-50 mIU/mL (mid-cycle peak)
- greater than 50 mIU/mL (postmenopausal)

Lactate dehydrogenase, serum: 140-280 U/L

Osmolality, serum: 280-300 mOsm/kg H_2O

Oxygen saturation, arterial blood: 95 % or greater

Phosphatase (alkaline), serum: 30-120 U/L

Phosphorus, serum: 3.0-4.5 mg/dL

Potassium, serum: 3.5-5.0 mEq/L

Triglycerides, serum (fasting)

- Normal: less than 250 mg/dL
- Borderline: 250-500 mg/dL
- Abnormal: greater than 500 mg/d

How to Overcome Test Anxiety

Just the thought of taking a test is enough to make most people a little nervous. A test is an important event that can have a long-term impact on your future, so it's important to take it seriously and it's natural to feel anxious about performing well. But just because anxiety is normal, that doesn't mean that it's helpful in test taking, or that you should simply accept it as part of your life. Anxiety can have a variety of effects. These effects can be mild, like making you feel slightly nervous, or severe, like blocking your ability to focus or remember even a simple detail.

If you experience test anxiety—whether severe or mild—it's important to know how to beat it. To discover this, first you need to understand what causes test anxiety.

Causes of Test Anxiety

While we often think of anxiety as an uncontrollable emotional state, it can actually be caused by simple, practical things. One of the most common causes of test anxiety is that a person does not feel adequately prepared for their test. This feeling can be the result of many different issues such as poor study habits or lack of organization, but the most common culprit is time management. Starting to study too late, failing to organize your study time to cover all of the material, or being distracted while you study will mean that you're not well prepared for the test. This may lead to cramming the night before, which will cause you to be physically and mentally exhausted for the test. Poor time management also contributes to feelings of stress, fear, and hopelessness as you realize you are not well prepared but don't know what to do about it.

Other times, test anxiety is not related to your preparation for the test but comes from unresolved fear. This may be a past failure on a test, or poor performance on tests in general. It may come from comparing yourself to others who seem to be performing better or from the stress of living up to expectations. Anxiety may be driven by fears of the future—how failure on this test would affect your educational and career goals. These fears are often completely irrational, but they can still negatively impact your test performance.

Review Video: 3 Reasons You Have Test Anxiety
Visit mometrix.com/academy and enter code: 428468

Elements of Test Anxiety

As mentioned earlier, test anxiety is considered to be an emotional state, but it has physical and mental components as well. Sometimes you may not even realize that you are suffering from test anxiety until you notice the physical symptoms. These can include trembling hands, rapid heartbeat, sweating, nausea, and tense muscles. Extreme anxiety may lead to fainting or vomiting. Obviously, any of these symptoms can have a negative impact on testing. It is important to recognize them as soon as they begin to occur so that you can address the problem before it damages your performance.

Review Video: 3 Ways to Tell You Have Test Anxiety
Visit mometrix.com/academy and enter code: 927847

The mental components of test anxiety include trouble focusing and inability to remember learned information. During a test, your mind is on high alert, which can help you recall information and stay focused for an extended period of time. However, anxiety interferes with your mind's natural processes, causing you to blank out, even on the questions you know well. The strain of testing during anxiety makes it difficult to stay focused, especially on a test that may take several hours. Extreme anxiety can take a huge mental toll, making it difficult not only to recall test information but even to understand the test questions or pull your thoughts together.

Review Video: How Test Anxiety Affects Memory
Visit mometrix.com/academy and enter code: 609003

Effects of Test Anxiety

Test anxiety is like a disease—if left untreated, it will get progressively worse. Anxiety leads to poor performance, and this reinforces the feelings of fear and failure, which in turn lead to poor performances on subsequent tests. It can grow from a mild nervousness to a crippling condition. If allowed to progress, test anxiety can have a big impact on your schooling, and consequently on your future.

Test anxiety can spread to other parts of your life. Anxiety on tests can become anxiety in any stressful situation, and blanking on a test can turn into panicking in a job situation. But fortunately, you don't have to let anxiety rule your testing and determine your grades. There are a number of relatively simple steps you can take to move past anxiety and function normally on a test and in the rest of life.

Review Video: How Test Anxiety Impacts Your Grades
Visit mometrix.com/academy and enter code: 939819

Physical Steps for Beating Test Anxiety

While test anxiety is a serious problem, the good news is that it can be overcome. It doesn't have to control your ability to think and remember information. While it may take time, you can begin taking steps today to beat anxiety.

Just as your first hint that you may be struggling with anxiety comes from the physical symptoms, the first step to treating it is also physical. Rest is crucial for having a clear, strong mind. If you are tired, it is much easier to give in to anxiety. But if you establish good sleep habits, your body and mind will be ready to perform optimally, without the strain of exhaustion. Additionally, sleeping well helps you to retain information better, so you're more likely to recall the answers when you see the test questions.

Getting good sleep means more than going to bed on time. It's important to allow your brain time to relax. Take study breaks from time to time so it doesn't get overworked, and don't study right before bed. Take time to rest your mind before trying to rest your body, or you may find it difficult to fall asleep.

Review Video: The Importance of Sleep for Your Brain
Visit mometrix.com/academy and enter code: 319338

Along with sleep, other aspects of physical health are important in preparing for a test. Good nutrition is vital for good brain function. Sugary foods and drinks may give a burst of energy but this burst is followed by a crash, both physically and emotionally. Instead, fuel your body with protein and vitamin-rich foods.

Also, drink plenty of water. Dehydration can lead to headaches and exhaustion, especially if your brain is already under stress from the rigors of the test. Particularly if your test is a long one, drink water during the breaks. And if possible, take an energy-boosting snack to eat between sections.

Review Video: How Diet Can Affect your Mood
Visit mometrix.com/academy and enter code: 624317

Along with sleep and diet, a third important part of physical health is exercise. Maintaining a steady workout schedule is helpful, but even taking 5-minute study breaks to walk can help get your blood pumping faster and clear your head. Exercise also releases endorphins, which contribute to a positive feeling and can help combat test anxiety.

When you nurture your physical health, you are also contributing to your mental health. If your body is healthy, your mind is much more likely to be healthy as well. So take time to rest, nourish your body with healthy food and water, and get moving as much as possible. Taking these physical steps will make you stronger and more able to take the mental steps necessary to overcome test anxiety.

Review Video: How to Stay Healthy and Prevent Test Anxiety
Visit mometrix.com/academy and enter code: 877894

Mental Steps for Beating Test Anxiety

Working on the mental side of test anxiety can be more challenging, but as with the physical side, there are clear steps you can take to overcome it. As mentioned earlier, test anxiety often stems from lack of preparation, so the obvious solution is to prepare for the test. Effective studying may be the most important weapon you have for beating test anxiety, but you can and should employ several other mental tools to combat fear.

First, boost your confidence by reminding yourself of past success—tests or projects that you aced. If you're putting as much effort into preparing for this test as you did for those, there's no reason you should expect to fail here. Work hard to prepare; then trust your preparation.

Second, surround yourself with encouraging people. It can be helpful to find a study group, but be sure that the people you're around will encourage a positive attitude. If you spend time with others who are anxious or cynical, this will only contribute to your own anxiety. Look for others who are motivated to study hard from a desire to succeed, not from a fear of failure.

Third, reward yourself. A test is physically and mentally tiring, even without anxiety, and it can be helpful to have something to look forward to. Plan an activity following the test, regardless of the outcome, such as going to a movie or getting ice cream.

When you are taking the test, if you find yourself beginning to feel anxious, remind yourself that you know the material. Visualize successfully completing the test. Then take a few deep, relaxing breaths and return to it. Work through the questions carefully but with confidence, knowing that you are capable of succeeding.

Developing a healthy mental approach to test taking will also aid in other areas of life. Test anxiety affects more than just the actual test—it can be damaging to your mental health and even contribute to depression. It's important to beat test anxiety before it becomes a problem for more than testing.

Review Video: Test Anxiety and Depression
Visit mometrix.com/academy and enter code: 904704

Study Strategy

Being prepared for the test is necessary to combat anxiety, but what does being prepared look like? You may study for hours on end and still not feel prepared. What you need is a strategy for test prep. The next few pages outline our recommended steps to help you plan out and conquer the challenge of preparation.

Step 1: Scope Out the Test

Learn everything you can about the format (multiple choice, essay, etc.) and what will be on the test. Gather any study materials, course outlines, or sample exams that may be available. Not only will this help you to prepare, but knowing what to expect can help to alleviate test anxiety.

Step 2: Map Out the Material

Look through the textbook or study guide and make note of how many chapters or sections it has. Then divide these over the time you have. For example, if a book has 15 chapters and you have five days to study, you need to cover three chapters each day. Even better, if you have the time, leave an extra day at the end for overall review after you have gone through the material in depth.

If time is limited, you may need to prioritize the material. Look through it and make note of which sections you think you already have a good grasp on, and which need review. While you are studying, skim quickly through the familiar sections and take more time on the challenging parts. Write out your plan so you don't get lost as you go. Having a written plan also helps you feel more in control of the study, so anxiety is less likely to arise from feeling overwhelmed at the amount to cover.

Step 3: Gather Your Tools

Decide what study method works best for you. Do you prefer to highlight in the book as you study and then go back over the highlighted portions? Or do you type out notes of the important information? Or is it helpful to make flashcards that you can carry with you? Assemble the pens, index cards, highlighters, post-it notes, and any other materials you may need so you won't be distracted by getting up to find things while you study.

If you're having a hard time retaining the information or organizing your notes, experiment with different methods. For example, try color-coding by subject with colored pens, highlighters, or post-it notes. If you learn better by hearing, try recording yourself reading your notes so you can listen while in the car, working out, or simply sitting at your desk. Ask a friend to quiz you from your flashcards, or try teaching someone the material to solidify it in your mind.

Step 4: Create Your Environment

It's important to avoid distractions while you study. This includes both the obvious distractions like visitors and the subtle distractions like an uncomfortable chair (or a too-comfortable couch that makes you want to fall asleep). Set up the best study environment possible: good lighting and a comfortable work area. If background music helps you focus, you may want to turn it on, but otherwise keep the room quiet. If you are using a computer to take notes, be sure you don't have any other windows open, especially applications like social media, games, or anything else that could distract you. Silence your phone and turn off notifications. Be sure to keep water close by so you stay hydrated while you study (but avoid unhealthy drinks and snacks).

Also, take into account the best time of day to study. Are you freshest first thing in the morning? Try to set aside some time then to work through the material. Is your mind clearer in the afternoon or evening? Schedule your study session then. Another method is to study at the same time of day that you will take the test, so that your brain gets used to working on the material at that time and will be ready to focus at test time.

STEP 5: STUDY!

Once you have done all the study preparation, it's time to settle into the actual studying. Sit down, take a few moments to settle your mind so you can focus, and begin to follow your study plan. Don't give in to distractions or let yourself procrastinate. This is your time to prepare so you'll be ready to fearlessly approach the test. Make the most of the time and stay focused.

Of course, you don't want to burn out. If you study too long you may find that you're not retaining the information very well. Take regular study breaks. For example, taking five minutes out of every hour to walk briskly, breathing deeply and swinging your arms, can help your mind stay fresh.

As you get to the end of each chapter or section, it's a good idea to do a quick review. Remind yourself of what you learned and work on any difficult parts. When you feel that you've mastered the material, move on to the next part. At the end of your study session, briefly skim through your notes again.

But while review is helpful, cramming last minute is NOT. If at all possible, work ahead so that you won't need to fit all your study into the last day. Cramming overloads your brain with more information than it can process and retain, and your tired mind may struggle to recall even previously learned information when it is overwhelmed with last-minute study. Also, the urgent nature of cramming and the stress placed on your brain contribute to anxiety. You'll be more likely to go to the test feeling unprepared and having trouble thinking clearly.

So don't cram, and don't stay up late before the test, even just to review your notes at a leisurely pace. Your brain needs rest more than it needs to go over the information again. In fact, plan to finish your studies by noon or early afternoon the day before the test. Give your brain the rest of the day to relax or focus on other things, and get a good night's sleep. Then you will be fresh for the test and better able to recall what you've studied.

STEP 6: TAKE A PRACTICE TEST

Many courses offer sample tests, either online or in the study materials. This is an excellent resource to check whether you have mastered the material, as well as to prepare for the test format and environment.

Check the test format ahead of time: the number of questions, the type (multiple choice, free response, etc.), and the time limit. Then create a plan for working through them. For example, if you have 30 minutes to take a 60-question test, your limit is 30 seconds per question. Spend less time on the questions you know well so that you can take more time on the difficult ones.

If you have time to take several practice tests, take the first one open book, with no time limit. Work through the questions at your own pace and make sure you fully understand them. Gradually work up to taking a test under test conditions: sit at a desk with all study materials put away and set a timer. Pace yourself to make sure you finish the test with time to spare and go back to check your answers if you have time.

After each test, check your answers. On the questions you missed, be sure you understand why you missed them. Did you misread the question (tests can use tricky wording)? Did you forget the information? Or was it something you hadn't learned? Go back and study any shaky areas that the practice tests reveal.

Taking these tests not only helps with your grade, but also aids in combating test anxiety. If you're already used to the test conditions, you're less likely to worry about it, and working through tests until you're scoring well gives you a confidence boost. Go through the practice tests until you feel comfortable, and then you can go into the test knowing that you're ready for it.

Test Tips

On test day, you should be confident, knowing that you've prepared well and are ready to answer the questions. But aside from preparation, there are several test day strategies you can employ to maximize your performance.

First, as stated before, get a good night's sleep the night before the test (and for several nights before that, if possible). Go into the test with a fresh, alert mind rather than staying up late to study.

Try not to change too much about your normal routine on the day of the test. It's important to eat a nutritious breakfast, but if you normally don't eat breakfast at all, consider eating just a protein bar. If you're a coffee drinker, go ahead and have your normal coffee. Just make sure you time it so that the caffeine doesn't wear off right in the middle of your test. Avoid sugary beverages, and drink enough water to stay hydrated but not so much that you need a restroom break 10 minutes into the test. If your test isn't first thing in the morning, consider going for a walk or doing a light workout before the test to get your blood flowing.

Allow yourself enough time to get ready, and leave for the test with plenty of time to spare so you won't have the anxiety of scrambling to arrive in time. Another reason to be early is to select a good seat. It's helpful to sit away from doors and windows, which can be distracting. Find a good seat, get out your supplies, and settle your mind before the test begins.

When the test begins, start by going over the instructions carefully, even if you already know what to expect. Make sure you avoid any careless mistakes by following the directions.

Then begin working through the questions, pacing yourself as you've practiced. If you're not sure on an answer, don't spend too much time on it, and don't let it shake your confidence. Either skip it and come back later, or eliminate as many wrong answers as possible and guess among the remaining ones. Don't dwell on these questions as you continue—put them out of your mind and focus on what lies ahead.

Be sure to read all of the answer choices, even if you're sure the first one is the right answer. Sometimes you'll find a better one if you keep reading. But don't second-guess yourself if you do immediately know the answer. Your gut instinct is usually right. Don't let test anxiety rob you of the information you know.

If you have time at the end of the test (and if the test format allows), go back and review your answers. Be cautious about changing any, since your first instinct tends to be correct, but make sure you didn't misread any of the questions or accidentally mark the wrong answer choice. Look over any you skipped and make an educated guess.

At the end, leave the test feeling confident. You've done your best, so don't waste time worrying about your performance or wishing you could change anything. Instead, celebrate the successful completion of this test. And finally, use this test to learn how to deal with anxiety even better next time.

Review Video: 5 Tips to Beat Test Anxiety
Visit mometrix.com/academy and enter code: 570656

Important Qualification

Not all anxiety is created equal. If your test anxiety is causing major issues in your life beyond the classroom or testing center, or if you are experiencing troubling physical symptoms related to your anxiety, it may be a sign of a serious physiological or psychological condition. If this sounds like your situation, we strongly encourage you to seek professional help.

Thank You

We at Mometrix would like to extend our heartfelt thanks to you, our friend and patron, for allowing us to play a part in your journey. It is a privilege to serve people from all walks of life who are unified in their commitment to building the best future they can for themselves.

The preparation you devote to these important testing milestones may be the most valuable educational opportunity you have for making a real difference in your life. We encourage you to put your heart into it—that feeling of succeeding, overcoming, and yes, conquering will be well worth the hours you've invested.

We want to hear your story, your struggles and your successes, and if you see any opportunities for us to improve our materials so we can help others even more effectively in the future, please share that with us as well. **The team at Mometrix would be absolutely thrilled to hear from you!** So please, send us an email (support@mometrix.com) and let's stay in touch.

If you'd like some additional help, check out these other resources we offer for your exam: http://MometrixFlashcards.com/RD

Additional Bonus Material

Due to our efforts to try to keep this book to a manageable length, we've created a link that will give you access to all of your additional bonus material.

Please visit http://www.mometrix.com/bonus948/rd to access the information.

CPSIA information can be obtained
at www.ICGtesting.com
Printed in the USA
LVHW060829020621
689128LV00003B/78